MORE THAN YOU CAN SEE

MORE THAN YOU CAN SEE

A Mother's Memoir

BARBARA RUBIN

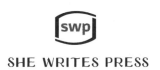

SHE WRITES PRESS

Published 2022
Printed in the United States of America
Print ISBN: 978-1-64742-249-3
E-ISBN: 978-1-64742-250-9
Library of Congress Control Number: 2022906754

For information, address:
She Writes Press
1569 Solano Ave #546
Berkeley, CA 94707

Interior design by Tabitha Lahr

She Writes Press is a division of SparkPoint Studio, LLC.

Names and identifying characteristics have been changed to protect the privacy of certain individuals.

Interior photos are from the author's personal archive.

To my husband, Mark,
who is the glue that holds me together.

Chapter 1

THE ACCIDENT

So beautiful and peaceful was that bright summer's day of July 1, 1991, when our lives were forever changed. My husband, Mark, and I were sitting on our deck looking out over the backyard that bordered woods as we reflected on the rewards of raising our daughters, Amy, thirteen, and Jenn, seventeen. There wasn't often time as a parent to stop and evaluate where you were in life; busy schedules keep everyone on the go at a frantic pace. But that afternoon, there was a brief pause in our busyness to talk about all we had accomplished. Finances had reached a stable point. We owned our home in a kid-friendly neighborhood, and I'd started working part-time as an accountant, setting my own hours while the girls were in school. We were seeing what amazing people our children were growing up to be. Both girls were good students and well accepted socially. They were kindhearted, honest, and trustworthy. Ours was a loving family of two parents, two beautiful girls, and two Siamese cats. That afternoon, everything seemed perfect.

The phone rang; I ran into the kitchen to answer it. Amy was home in her room, but Jenn was off with friends. Whenever our girls were out of the house, I couldn't let a call go unanswered.

"This is St. Luke's hospital calling. There was a car accident, and your daughter has been admitted to the hospital. You should come right away," said the woman's voice on the other end of the line. I started screaming from the kitchen to Mark who was still on the deck, "There's been an accident, we have to go." I was frantic, scrambling to get my shoes on as he grabbed the keys, and we headed out the door. We raced to the hospital emergency room, my heart pounding. I was still hopeful that Jenn's injuries would be minor.

We identified ourselves to the lady at the registration desk, and someone led us into a private office where a nurse with a serious face began explaining the extent of Jenn's injuries. "Your daughter is unconscious and in critical condition. She has various injuries but most serious is the one to her head."

I couldn't breathe. Was this really happening?

The nurse went on. "I'll take you in to see her now. Doctors will be in shortly to further brief you on the details."

This was a nightmare: My daughter was not just hurt, she was in critical condition. I didn't want too many details. I just wanted to see her.

I'd never witnessed a person in critical condition, so I was unprepared for the sight awaiting me as I entered Jenn's room. Machines monitored her heart rate and pulse. Tubes were hanging from various parts of her body. My beautiful daughter's face was severely bruised, and her flawless skin was swollen. Her cascading blonde hair was matted with blood, and there was a nasty cut on one of her eyebrows above her closed eyes. Blood seeped through bandages on her right hand. Her breathing was shallow, and the only movement I could see was the slight rise and fall of her chest beneath her gown.

That was too much for me to take in. I moved forward in slow motion, each step affirming the reality of this terrible trauma. The only sound I heard was the beeping of monitors. In my mind, the ten steps it took to be by Jenn's side stretched into a long corridor of void as I approached her bedside. All I wanted to do was touch her, hold her, and make all the bad go away.

We had only a few moments alone with our daughter before doctors arrived to explain that Jenn had suffered a traumatic brain injury and was in a deep coma. I began to understand that her life was a fragile step away from death.

THE AFTERNOON HOURS slipped away and, as the late evening approached, Jenn was moved to an ICU room where we began our vigil over her. Beeping monitors and the continuous flow of doctors and nurses kept us alert for any change that would signal a turn for the worse. The medical staff could not offer anything other than the fact that she was alive. Mark and I clung to each other, our faces saying more than words ever could.

Within twenty-four hours of the impact, Jenn's brain began to swell, causing even further damage. Blood rushed to her brain, the body's way of preserving its most precious organ. On the second day after a long night at her bedside, her neurosurgeon told us, "Your daughter needs brain surgery to relieve the pressure in her skull."

The words "brain surgery" were crushing—it sounded more like a death sentence than a way to save my daughter's life. "Oh, my God, is there any way to avoid this?" I asked as tears flowed down my cheeks.

"No, her life depends on this surgery, and every moment we delay, more damage is taking place. She also needs to be put on a ventilator to help with her breathing; this will be done at the same time. The risks are great that she might not survive the surgery, but doing nothing would be a grave mistake." We read the urgency of the situation in his words and the sad sullen expression on his face.

With no other choice, Mark and I signed a release for the procedures. The doctor grabbed the document, directed the nursing staff to take us to the surgical waiting room, and then quickly disappeared down the hall to the operating room.

We huddled in the waiting room clinging to each other as we watched the hands on the wall clock tick slowly by. "It's horrible not to know how the surgery is going," Mark whispered.

"It's taking so long," I whispered back a short time later. I looked at my watch—we'd been waiting an hour. I felt wretched; my stomach seemed to be lodged in my throat. They'd told us it would take two hours, but as the minutes ticked by, I began to feel physically ill. The stress of the past twenty-four hours weighed heavily on my mind and body. I felt ready to collapse. A nurse came in to check on us and bring us some snacks. Something about my demeanor must have alarmed her. She sat on the sofa next to me and took my vitals. Assured that I wasn't going to pass out, she walked out of the room, leaving Mark and me with food we had no appetite for and a silence that was deafening.

I was trying to deal with overwhelming anxiety, but as I looked at Mark sitting next to me, I was comforted by his presence. My loving and tender husband, who was in so many ways my better half, was suffering just as much as I was. It was written all over his face—eyes downcast, mouth tightly drawn. A new line of despair creased his brow. Stubble from his beard was beginning to appear on his face. His dark curly hair was uncombed. My handsome warrior was shaken, and his facade of physical strength showed cracks. I reached for his hand which was always available for me to hold and gave it a squeeze—my way of saying, *We'll get through this, somehow.*

After what seemed like an eternity, the doctor came to tell us that Jenn was in the recovery room. At last, we could take a deep breath.

"Your daughter did well through the surgery, but she's in critical condition. It's watch and wait for the next few hours."

The surgeon explained that a three-inch-diameter piece of her skull had been removed to drain the bleed and then put back in place. "If this doesn't relieve the pressure, I will have to drill holes in her skull to allow the brain to protrude through them until that swelling goes down."

He also explained about a brain monitor that he implanted into the base of her skull to track the swelling. We listened and exchanged worried glances. It all sounded terrifying.

After another hour, Jenn was moved back to the ICU, and we returned to her bedside. To see her again and know that she was still with us brought another flood of emotions. Mark and I held each other as we stood watching the brain monitor screen and praying for God to spare her life and let us keep our daughter. Neither of us wanted to leave her side as we patiently waited through the night, her beeping monitors our only comfort, as they assured us she was still alive.

DURING THE COURSE of the past thirty hours, neither Mark nor I had returned home. We knew we needed to make contact with our daughter Amy, so we called her from the payphone down the hall from Jenn's room in the ICU. Mark did the talking as I couldn't hold my emotions in check long enough to get any words out. We didn't want to scare Amy unnecessarily, but we knew that she had to be told enough to help her understand the situation was serious.

I listened in as Mark called her. "Amy, how are you doing?"

"I'm okay dad. Cara is here with me, but how is Jenn?"

"Well, it's serious, really serious. Your sister is unconscious and in a coma. One of her fingers is in bad shape and needs surgery in the coming days, but for now, they want to let her recover a bit more before doing that. Mom is here beside me and sends her love. We don't know when we will get home so call the neighbors if you need anything."

"No worries, Dad, I'll be fine. Stay with Jenn and let me know if anything changes."

It was not surprising that Amy was so composed. Independent from the time she could walk, our petite, younger daughter was always confident and, throughout her short thirteen years, had shown us she was more than capable of taking care of herself. Wise beyond her years, she was sweet and lovable but not someone who could be taken advantage of because of her size. Her less than five-foot frame disguised the powerhouse personality that resided in her small body. Unlike her sister who was five-six, Amy was petite and not likely to catch up to her sister in height.

We didn't press Amy to come to the hospital. We felt Jenn's condition was too distressing for her to see. Amy was strong, but we didn't want her to see her parents so emotionally shattered. We suggested she wait a few days before visiting her sister.

TWO DAYS AFTER the accident, the hospital called us into the business office and said we would need a lawyer. Expenses were accumulating and we had already exhausted any accidental insurance coverage. Really? We had to deal with this too, money and bills, when all we wanted was to be with our daughter?

Thankfully, I knew of a legal firm who could represent us and gave them a call. One of the attorneys from the firm, Marc, came to the hospital almost immediately to gather information. Once the legal team was in place, we were never questioned or harassed about the rapidly mounting medical bills. The law firm gave us the liberty to deal solely with the crisis of our daughter's injuries.

Marc came to the hospital often to consult with us and to check on Jenn's condition. Like us, he was in his early forties, sporting dark hair that had yet to see any touches of gray. From the first time he came to the hospital, I felt he connected with us emotionally and professionally. He seemed to truly care about us and our daughter.

It was through him that we learned the details of what had happened in the accident. The most significant information he gave was that the other vehicle was a cement truck, and that driver was at fault, causing the accident. "Tire marks show the truck was in the middle of the roadway and speeding," he explained. "We are going to file a lawsuit immediately against the cement company. We also need to file suit against the young driver of the vehicle where Jenn was a passenger to have access to her liability coverage."

Marc explained more of the situation to us: "Here are some of the facts as I know them. The day of the accident presented no adverse weather conditions to obstruct the visibility of either driver. The accident happened on Toleman

Road at the tight curve with a slight incline just north of Washingtonville. Drivers have to use extra caution to successfully navigate that section of the road because they can't see traffic approaching from the other side until the last few seconds when they come to the top of the hill."

My husband and I knew the exact section he referred to. It was poorly designed to handle the constant flow of traffic that had come with the influx of development in Orange County, New York.

Marc continued, "With the truck straddling the middle of the narrow roadway, Jenn's driver had few options. Straight ahead was the truck. On her right and just next to the outer part of the curve was a fence and a house five feet from the edge of the asphalt. On her left was a shoulder embankment—she went left, away from the truck barreling down on her, but that put Jenn in peril. The truck slammed into the passenger side, and the high off-road bumper crushed the roof of the car into Jenn's head.

"When the rescue teams arrived, they found the truck driver uninjured. Jenn's driver had a severely broken arm and was in shock, leaving her unable to identify Jenn, who was unconscious and pinned inside the crushed car. They had to extract Jenn from the vehicle using the jaws of life before taking her by ambulance to the hospital.

"The police report indicates the truck driver was at fault. It's an ongoing investigation, and I will fill you in on other details as they come to light."

As Marc talked about the accident, images of Jenn crushed in the car flashed into my mind and were beyond painful to process. But hearing his words placing guilt clearly on the truck driver stirred a new emotional response in me—rage!

I knew one thing for certain, I didn't want anything to

do with the truck driver. I alerted hospital staff and Marc to keep the truck driver from coming near us. "We want no notes, no visits, no contact. We don't want to know his name or what he looks like."

I was so enraged with this driver I couldn't bear to have his image permanently implanted in my mind. I didn't want to see this person out in public at the grocery store, mall, or on the street and be reminded of what he'd done to our daughter.

IT WAS PAINFUL FOR us to hear the circumstances of the accident that put Jenn in harm's way. We knew that she and her friends were taking an exchange student class-mate to the Newark Airport for a return flight to her home in Spain. Jenn, Rachael, and Jenn's boyfriend, Greg, were headed home afterward. Marc filled us in on the scenario: "They'd dropped Greg off at his house, leaving the two girls traveling alone on the narrow winding country road back to your home, and then the worst thing imaginable happened."

Jenn's reaction to the impending collision must have been to put her hand over her face—we could see the evidence clearly on the hand she used to cover her right eye. Her ring finger was crushed, and plastic shards from the mangled dashboard had pierced her hand in various places.

The finger required surgery by a hand specialist to repair it as much as possible, but this procedure was delayed until a week after the accident when her condition was less fragile. The ring she wore and the finger structure helped to absorb some of the impact from the collision, perhaps even saving her life. But her head took such a hard blow that the bone structure around her right eye was fractured. The neurosurgeon told us that the orbital bones would heal on their own, "But important neurons were ripped apart as her brain smashed into her skull. The damage is significant and life-threatening," he told us, trying to put everything in perspective.

WORD ABOUT JENNIFER'S accident quickly spread throughout our community. Over the coming days, friends gathered by her bedside. Gifts of stuffed animals, cards, and flowers quickly filled the room with the loving support of those who cared deeply for her and our family.

Greg visited daily, usually bringing Amy with him. It was cute how over the course of his courtship with Jenn, he'd always treated her younger sibling as a little sister. At six feet tall, he towered over Amy. Mark and I absolutely loved this guy. He was soft-spoken with a gentle nature that perfectly matched Jenn's personality. When giving him a hug, you could feel his muscles, making it easy to guess that he spent hours working out with his weight-lifting equipment. He and Jenn were quite the handsome couple. Of course, I thought my daughter was a knockout, and Greg could have easily been a model with his thick, dark hair, strong brow, and deep-set eyes. What was far more important was that both were humble and personable, truly inclusive of all who were around them.

Jenn's friend Rachael, the driver, and her parents came a few times, but that ended after they learned we'd filed a lawsuit against them. I wished they hadn't taken it personally—it was simply a matter of securing the liability dollars held by their insurance company.

Two of Jenn's close girlfriends, Lisa and Jayme, were among the first visitors. They were surprised to hear that authorities were unable to identify Jenn at the scene of the collision. "Jenn didn't go anywhere without her purse, so why wasn't it found and her license used to identify her?" Lisa asked.

"Our lawyer said the authorities looked for it in the car and around the accident site, but it wasn't there," I explained.

"What? That's ridiculous. It has to be somewhere," Jayme added.

"We're going to look for it." Together they decided to help piece together more details about the accident by finding the purse. It meant a lot to us that they would do that.

The two girls went to the accident location and spent hours scouring the area, but like the police and firefighters, found nothing. If the purse wasn't at the accident site, then it had to be in the car. They went to the auto wreckage yard and began carefully searching the crushed vehicle. It turned up nothing, but they took on the search as a mission. Finally, their efforts paid off. They found Jenn's pocketbook wedged up under the dashboard. It had survived the crash, undetectable to others who didn't have the same determination to find it.

Retrieving the purse might seem like a small matter, but it took on a more meaningful role to me. This personal item represented who Jenn was before fate had put her in harm's way. As I held it, I was holding the daughter I had before the accident.

DURING THOSE INITIAL hospital days when Jenn was in critical condition, I was crushed with agony. It took superhuman effort to compose myself enough to eat, sleep, or put one foot in front of the other to get through my day. How could people continue to be happy and enjoy things when my whole world had come crashing down? My mind and body cried out for me to collapse into a useless bundle of flesh. But I knew I had to hold everything together to help rally my daughter, who was fighting for her life. I functioned marginally. My total focus was on Jennifer and getting her to live.

Life-support systems were in place. Jenn was on a ventilator, and a feeding tube was inserted into her abdomen. All this was done even as the hospital pressed us to sign a release form for Jenn's organs to be donated in the event of her death. Every day that she survived was a day we did not have to face the unthinkable. This intensity lasted for ten days as the coma persisted, and the outcome continued to be uncertain.

Neither Mark nor I spoke the word *death* out loud; it was too painful to even imagine. Instead, we tried to latch on to the simple things the hospital's physical therapist showed us to do to keep Jennifer as limber as possible.

"You can help stimulate her brain as well as keep her from stiffening up by moving any and every joint of her body. Take her legs and move them up and down, in and out. Flex her knees and wiggle her toes. Bend her elbows and fingers."

I loved this advice and took it to heart. From that point on, we were constantly moving Jenn and touching her. We encouraged her visitors to do the same. Working to preserve the range of motion in her limbs was a great distraction and made us feel we were doing something that could have a positive result.

After ten days, Jenn's eyes opened, and she slowly began to emerge from the darkness of her coma into a higher level of consciousness. She didn't respond to verbal commands like "squeeze my hand" or "blink your eyes," but she began to acknowledge sounds by turning her face toward them. With each passing hour and day, Jenn moved her hands and feet a bit more, and soon she was flailing around in her bed, her hands reaching to pull the tubes out of her body and picking at the bandages on her finger. We began to have hope. She was going to live, and we expected her recovery to bring her back to her original self, even as the neurosurgeon emphasized that it would be a slow process, and there would most likely be some disabilities resulting from her injury.

During the days Jenn was in a coma, it would have been easy for me to slip into a state of total despair. I teetered on the brink of sanity, but as quickly as dark thoughts came, I replaced them with the reminder that there was something bigger than myself at stake. At last, after all Jenn had gone through and the throes of death that she'd escaped, I had a daughter who was going to live. She would need me to help in her recovery. Our younger daughter, Amy, also still needed parenting and a family to help her—I knew that she too would be greatly affected by this tragedy. Life was moving on, and I needed to be engaged with everything that might unfold in the future.

Chapter 2

ON A NEW PATH

After a few gut-wrenching weeks of uncertainty, the doctors upgraded Jenn's condition from critical to stable. She was weaned off the ventilator, and hospital staff told us it was time to relocate her to a rehab facility. The best fit for someone with her low level of function was the Hillcrest Rehabilitation Center located in Milford, Pennsylvania, an hour's drive from our home in New York. They would help her relearn the basic life skills of eating, sitting, walking, and communicating. She still hadn't spoken a single coherent word since the accident, only muttered garbled sounds.

It was hard to see Jenn in such a greatly impaired state when she first went to Hillcrest. She seemed dazed, barely aware of her surroundings. With little control over her body, she was like a rag doll, unable to hold herself erect, and she made random, nonpurposeful movements with her arms and legs. Placed in a wheelchair with a large tray table on the front to keep her in a somewhat seated position, she flopped around or slumped to one side. A towel was clipped to her shirt to catch the drool that streamed from her gaping mouth. It was painful to see that she was unrecognizable as her former self.

Jenn was not following verbal commands, so a speech pathologist, Lori, was assigned to her. She was a darling woman, with short, curly, brown hair, a gentle nature, and soft voice. She'd had eighteen years of experience and looked forward to working with Jenn. What neither of us knew at the time was that all her hard-won experience would be tested to its limits by her new client.

Lori's sessions began immediately upon Jenn's arrival at the facility. We watched as she first tried to make eye contact with Jenn and get her to respond to simple commands. Holding Jenn's head in her hands, she said, "Jenn, look at me. Jenn, can you hold your head up?" Lori repeated these commands many times, but Jenn played no active part in the process and made no response. Other therapists faced similar challenges in trying to get her to follow their directives.

It was difficult and heartbreaking being around someone in a semiconscious state. It was as bizarre as it was frightening. She seemed to be suspended in limbo, swimming in the murky waters of her coma and still fighting to reach the surface. The Hillcrest staff tried to reassure me they had seen this before. They understood she was working her way to a higher level of function, and the stimulation that all of us were giving her would help her in this battle.

Jenn's right hand began to curl into a fist, and her right arm showed signs of atrophy as she held her arm tightly against her body. In occupational therapy, she was non-compliant. These sessions were all about being touched and seemed to be painful to her—she would jerk back or make a sound of distress as they worked on her range of motion. Her therapist, Donna, drew upon her youthful strength to treat her combative client. Even something as benign as having her hand held open to be measured for a splint set Jenn into a fit of rage. Yelling, and using all her extremities to try and free herself, Jenn showed a strength that wasn't apparent when she was slumped in her wheelchair. Donna also began stretching the tightened arm, wrist, and fingers. The sessions were painful to watch, as Jenn screamed and fought with all her strength. I knew her arm and hand needed the therapy, but it still brought tears to my eyes as I watched each session and silently grieved for the pain my daughter had to endure.

Physical therapists concerned themselves with Jenn's posture and a right foot that was flexing downward. Her ankle was tight, and like her arm and hand, needed to be stretched. She moaned and fought them too, but I could tell that her protests were not from pain but from annoyance at not wanting to be touched. They were also trying to show Jenn how to use her hands and feet to move her wheelchair. For some reason, she was slightly more cooperative with that part of the session.

SLOWLY OVER A few weeks' time, Jenn began to work her way out of the fog. No longer were her eyes glazed. We could see her concentrate on things taking place around her. Her movements became more purposeful, and she held her body erect. A tray was no longer needed to hold her in place, and she was starting to regain control over her arms and legs. The drooling was gone, and she began to make facial expressions, even happy ones like smiling.

Mark and I had been solely focused on Jenn for weeks, but the time had come for us to consider how the changes in our family's life were affecting our younger daughter, Amy. Although she gave no outward appearance of being depressed, as concerned parents, we thought she might be suppressing her emotions which could lead to problems in the future. We felt obligated to send her to a child psychiatrist to get a professional opinion about how she was handling our family situation. We didn't want to be remiss in attending to her mental well-being.

Although the talk therapy seemed to be a good idea, after a couple of sessions, Amy became disenchanted with the whole process.

"He keeps asking me if I have thoughts of killing myself, which I don't," she said. "He talked about someone in my condition to which I got mad and said, 'I don't have a condition. My sister was in an accident. That's not a condition.'"

It was clear she wanted to end the sessions. "I think he's stupid, and he isn't doing anything positive for me!"

With that in mind, and the confirmation from the psychiatrist that he detected nothing alarming, we discontinued the psychiatric visits. In fact, our Amy was incredibly resilient for a young person who'd seen such a harsh reality of life. We had no immediate family in the area, but she'd formed a strong reliance on both her own and Jenn's close friends for support. No doubt Amy's upbeat personality also propelled her in a positive direction. The comfort from those dedicated friends helped our thirteen-year-old Amy survive and continue to thrive as we moved forward with Jenn's recovery.

MARK WAS A teacher, so when the school year started for him and Amy, I continued to go to Hillcrest every day on my own. I wheeled Jenn to her various therapy sessions and tried to be a quiet observer, sitting off to the side so as not to disturb either her or the therapists. The staff often wanted to engage me in conversation, explaining what they were doing and why. I found it fascinating and appreciated the information they shared.

Because of the orbital fractures sustained in her accident, Jenn's right eye was slightly skewed outward. The in-house doctor told us this would give her double vision until her brain adjusted and compensated for the damage by eventually ignoring the signal it received from that eye. I didn't understand how efficiently her damaged brain would be able to accomplish this task, but I trusted he knew what he was talking about.

To help in this compensation process, nurses began covering Jenn's skewed right eye with an adhesive eye patch, forcing her brain to work with the left eye alone. Having a bandage placed over her eye didn't set Jenn off like other therapies did, but she immediately pulled off the offending eye-cover. The nurse would put it back on just to have her pull it off again and again. "No, Jenn, leave it alone," she instructed while holding Jenn's hand so she couldn't get to the patch. Now Jenn was mad; once again someone was touching her and trying to force her to do or not do something. She screeched and twisted to free herself. Once the nurse released her hold, Jenn left the patch on and seemed content to just not be touched anymore. But when she was out of the nurse's line of vision, Jenn ripped it off and discarded it in a trashcan. Sometimes she went farther down the corridor, dropping the patch on the floor, or hiding it behind another client's wheelchair or under the cushion of her own wheelchair. It was like a broken record throughout the day: putting the patch on, and Jenn taking it off.

Hillcrest also had a computer program designed to retrain the eyes to work together. Jenn looked amused playing on the computer, pushing the buttons or moving the curser around on the screen. It was never clear if the program helped her vision, but it seemed a fun reprieve for her from some of the other unpleasant things people were making her do. Jenn overcame whatever visual difficulties she may have had rather quickly and never displayed dizziness or fainted. She did have some episodes of car sickness when we took her on short outings during those first few weeks at Hillcrest, but they quickly subsided.

Now that Jenn was more alert, Lori's communication sessions took on a different role. It was important to see if Jenn understood what was being said to her and to find a way for her to express herself.

In one of the exercises, Lori held up three different colored cards in front of Jenn. "Give me the green card, Jenn."

Jenn grabbed one of the cards, rubbed it on her forehead and threw it to the side. Lori tried again, but Jenn's choices were random; she showed no understanding of having picked the correct color, if in fact she had.

"Jenn, put the card in my hand," Lori said as she held out her palm. Jenn showed no pattern of understanding. Again, she took a card, rubbed it on her face and discarded it.

Lori also started trying to help Jenn relearn how to talk. "Jenn, can you say 'ba,' say 'ba' Jenn."

Other than moaning, Jenn made no attempt to copy the sounds Lori made. Despite all her years of experience, Lori told us she was puzzled by her new client. "I never had a person who lacked both receptive and expressive language skills. It's always one or the other, not both. This is going to be interesting."

As a speech pathologist, Lori was also responsible for eating and swallowing skills. Jenn showed no interest in food or drink and would not allow anything to be brought near her mouth. In fact, eating became the most urgent thing for her to master, as her feeding tube was becoming problematic and needed to be removed.

How do you start teaching a person one of life's most basic instincts—eating? The standard procedure starts with giving them puréed foods, taking care to keep the client from choking. Learning to eat is complicated, requiring control of the tongue, moving food around in the mouth and down the throat. But first a client must open their mouth to let the food in.

Lori began by placing sour lollipops on Jenn's lips, testing to see if she would open her mouth to taste them. Very resistant to any oral contact, Jenn turned her head and clamped her mouth shut. Day after day, Lori tried to entice Jenn to open her mouth with different flavors of lollipops, but nothing worked.

During this time, Jenn had learned to skillfully maneuver herself up and down the hallways of the facility in her wheelchair. She roamed freely as if it were an adventure. She rediscovered everyday things like doorknobs, light switches, and the elevator call button. She seemed to study each new thing, touching it and carefully running her fingers over the surface to see what it might do. When she figured out how to use a light switch, she went up and down the hallways flipping them off and on, but no matter how many times she flipped a particular switch, when she left the area it was always in the off position—a lesson learned from her childhood—turn the lights off when you leave a room. She tested doorknobs and loved when she was able to open up a door and peek inside. The world seemed to be an entirely new and fascinating place to her.

One day as she wheeled by a nursing cart, the nurse handed her a lollipop. Everyone knew that the speech therapist was trying to get Jenn to start eating, but the usual routine was for Jenn to take the treat and then deposit it somewhere along her path as she rolled on down the hallway. But this time, Jenn willingly stuffed the lollipop into her mouth. Crunch, crunch, crunch, and it was gone, consumed in seconds by the girl who had wanted nothing to do with food up to that point.

Nursing immediately consulted with Lori to find out if it was safe for Jenn to do this. "Don't give her any more until I see her tomorrow and check out her ability to swallow," Lori instructed. Even her words of caution didn't dispel the excitement that rang throughout the facility as everyone recognized the huge step forward Jenn had taken in her recovery by eating something—anything.

In Lori's next session, she and I watched as Jenn quickly consumed lollipops as soon as they were handed to her. After Jenn's first taste of the sweet round ball on a white stick, she seemed to know what it was and eagerly accepted any that were offered. "It's pretty obvious that she doesn't have a problem with swallowing," Lori confirmed.

But lollipops do not a balanced diet make. Lori moved her next session to the dining room for more space and easy access to the kitchen. New foods were offered—the puréed kind normally used to reintroduce a client to eating. But Jenn clamped her mouth shut and turned her face away from the offending muck. Lori quickly concluded that a whole new approach would be needed to teach her resistant client to eat something other than lollipops.

"Bring me some Cheerios," Lori called to the kitchen staff. "Let's see if they work," she laughingly said to me as I sat watching the session.

Taking a single Cheerio, Lori held it up for Jenn to see. "Eat, Jenn," she said before putting the Cheerio in her own mouth. Then she tried to take Jenn's hand and put a Cheerio in it but made the cardinal mistake of touching her and trying to force her to do something. Jenn's facial expressions were very animated by now, and she employed them to send a clear message where words evaded her. She leaned forward, got right in Lori's face and with a scornful look loudly groaned at her and quickly tucked her hand down into her lap.

"Okay, okay Jenn, I get it. I won't touch you. You do it."

With that Lori picked up another Cheerio and put it in her own mouth. She then pointed at one on the table and said, "Eat, Jenn."

After a couple of tries, Jenn picked up a Cheerio, put it in her mouth, chewed and swallowed it. She then gave Lori a little smirk as if to say, "Look who's in control here," or that was the way Lori and I interpreted it. We both started laughing and, to our added delight and surprise, Jenn joined in with us.

Had I really just laughed? It was a new feeling, something I hadn't done in months.

The session continued with Lori having a Cheerio, then offering Jenn one. But not all of Jenn's morsels ended up in her mouth. Some went in while others were dropped on the floor. Leaning over the side of her chair, she seemed fascinated by dropping them and watching them fall. Was she calculating the distance? Was she wondering how to get them back? I couldn't tell, but for some reason, one of every two or three Cheerios had to be dropped. Then unexpectedly, she winged one right at Lori, hitting her in the glasses.

Of course, Lori had a startled response, which Jenn apparently thought was hilarious as she broke out laughing. Lori tried to keep her composure to not let Jenn see the laugh she was holding back and hoping wouldn't escape from her lips. In a soft but stern voice and with a wagging finger, Lori tried to correct her. "No Jenn, no throwing."

That wagging finger was too much of a temptation for Jenn, she leaned forward with her mouth open as though she were going to bite it. Jenn was known to have bitten people recently; she had gotten me a few times. The attendants who took care of her daily hygiene were the main victims of this oral defense system Jenn used to keep people from doing things to her like brushing her teeth or combing her hair.

Knowing about the biting, Lori quickly withdrew her finger, but from Jenn's expression, I don't think biting was really her intension. I'm not sure what she might have done, but she was in a playful mood, so I don't think she was going to be vengeful.

As the days rolled ahead, it was fun to watch as Jenn became more willing to open her mouth and try the new foods Lori offered her. But if they were soft in texture, she quickly spit them out. When given a spoonful of ice cream, she left her mouth open, tongue out, and let the yucky stuff melt and drip off the end. Mashed potatoes must have felt nasty, as they were violently spit out, fortunately to the side and not at Lori. Raw vegetables were easily consumed, but meat was rejected. Hard and crunchy options were the only foods that she tolerated.

Lori also had to teach Jenn how to feed herself, which meant the dining room began to look like a school cafeteria after a food fight. Rejects became missiles of flying food globs. At times, it seemed Jenn even took careful aim and made people targets for the utensil or food item she was trying to launch as far away as possible.

Slowly, foods became tolerable, and in a relatively short time Jenn went from needing a feeding tube for all her nourishment to eating anything and everything she could get her hands on. *Everything!* She even tasted some nonedibles, like the crayons, pens, and the watch that we had her wear. Oops! Jenn didn't seem to be able to distinguish food from other objects that came into her range. Fortunately, this phase passed quickly, as it was a scary safety issue. But it did help me recognize just how foreign the world was to my daughter. She had to learn even the simplest of things like determining what was food and what wasn't.

IT WAS TIME to start helping Jenn relearn how to stand and walk. But, unfortunately, the physical therapy room must have looked like a torture chamber to her—she wedged herself in the doorway using her outstretched arms and legs to resist being pushed through the opening. It took two people to untangle her from the doorway and successfully usher her into the large well-equipped therapy room. Once inside, the therapist helped her to lay on a table before strapping her down. The table lifted her upright and held her in a standing position for several minutes. This treatment helped Jenn adjust to the upright stance and feel her body weight on her legs. Once the table was upright, Jenn seemed to relax, and a smile would come to her face. In a matter of a few weeks, they had her try walking.

Standing behind Jenn's wheelchair, I watched as two staff members, one on each side, helped Jenn to her feet. With one steadying her, the other therapist lifted each leg and placed it on the floor. It was an exciting moment to witness her first steps, and I cheered her on, encouraging her with a round of applause. My response seemed to have a positive effect on her willingness to work with the therapists. Perhaps it reassured her, as she became more compliant and allowed them to manipulate her legs and feet.

Because of the injury, Jenn was prone to toe walking. Rather than placing her heel down at the start of each step, Jenn instead put her toes on the floor first, particularly with her right foot. By repeated correct foot placement, the therapists worked to reprogram Jenn's brain in proper gait movement. Within days, with the help of an assistant holding her steady, she was moving her legs on her own—not perfectly, but with purpose. Squeals from a happy Jenn echoed around the room as she seemed to recognize that she was gaining a new control over her body. She seemed eager to keep learning this new walking thing.

Several times a day, an assistant would help Jenn out of her wheelchair and, using a PT belt secured around Jenn's waist, would walk her up and down the hallways. The physical therapist was trying to hold Jenn back from walking alone until her gait was right, but after many weeks of training, it was clear that wasn't going to happen. So, to prevent Jenn from toe walking with her right foot, she fitted her with an ankle brace that didn't allow the ankle to flex, therefore not letting the toes down before the heel. Jenn was tolerant of the brace, had the strength to walk on her own, and showed that she had no balance issues. So the therapist gave her approval for Jenn to be allowed to ambulate independently. At last, Jenn was free of her wheelchair.

With the new mobility, we were able to bring her home on some Saturdays for an overnight. Walking Jenn into the house that first time was monumental. She needed assistance navigating the steps along the driveway, at the front porch, and up the short flight once inside the house. But with Mark on one side and me on the other, she was easy to help.

It was wonderful but exhausting to have her home. Mark slept on the floor in her room to be sure she wasn't getting up or didn't fall out of bed during the night. Throughout the day, she required constant supervision and interaction. Sitting her on the living room floor, we brought out old toys from her childhood that we hadn't yet disposed of and let her rediscover the noises they made and the way they felt. She particularly liked opening containers and finding small treasures inside. We liked keeping her stimulated and entertained. Her curiosity as she checked out each item was reminiscent of the reaction our kids had as toddlers—but this realization was both sobering and encouraging. We knew her curiosity would move her forward in recovery, but it was still hard to see how regressed she really was.

The six-inch-square wooden box that she and Dad made in the garage when she was a kid was a favorite. She opened the metal clasp without a problem and was quick to dump out the random items we put inside. She laughed and smiled as she picked each thing up. The small spongy ball was given a squeeze, a shake, and tossed aside. The Lincoln Log was of little interest and was quickly discarded. She didn't like the playing cards either until Mark flicked one up in the air, which she found hysterical. She picked up one and success- fully mimicked him by flicking it a short distance. She eagerly engaged in this newfound activity and began flicking cards all over the place. She seemed fascinated to see how far she could propel them. Her dexterity to carefully fold each card just the right amount to launch it in the air astounded us.

We were challenged to find new activities and things for her to explore. Amy liked playing mini basketball with her sister. A small hoop was hooked on the back of a kitchen chair making it reachable from the floor or sofa. The soft padded ball would do no harm if Jenn decided to throw it at a lamp or person. The girls would take turns throwing the ball at the basket, sometimes even getting it in. Amy had to do all the retrieving and Jenn liked taking more than her fair share of turns. But we could see that Amy was thrilled just to be able to get Jenn to smile or laugh; she wasn't concerned about turns.

Friends often came to visit when Jenn was home, especially Greg. He would sit on the floor with her and fling cards at a target, roll balls back and forth, or hand her pieces of a wooden puzzle for her to assemble. Jenn was happy to interact with him or other friends when they came; she smiled, laughed, and giggled, but there didn't appear to be any special recognition of these people. Her reaction to them was no different from her reaction to the therapists at Hillcrest.

Come Sunday morning, we drove Jenn back to Hillcrest where we would spend the day with her as a family.

THE MILFORD PLACEMENT was not only a healing place for Jenn, but also for Mark, Amy, and me. We were surrounded by other suffering families who understood that a good day didn't mean everything was going to be all better. We all knew that one small step in recovery by anyone's family member was significant and was celebrated as a notable accomplishment by everyone there. Bad days came too: seizures, behavior outbursts, additional surgeries, infections, and questions, always questions: Where does all this lead?

Little did I know that, as a result of the time we spent in this unique environment, Amy's life would find direction that would serve as a guiding force in her future. She watched how the therapists broke down everyday tasks into simple steps so the client could relearn each part of a skill. Something as mundane as using a fork to eat was made up of many separate and sequential actions that these clients no longer remembered: which hand to use, which end of the fork goes into the food, how to pick up a food item with this utensil, how to bring it into the mouth, and finally how to make the lips pull food off the fork. "I love the way therapists break down everyday tasks to teach these people how to do things," she told us. "If they can't learn a skill, it gets broken down into even smaller steps."

Amy repeatedly told us that watching the problem-solving used in rehab was interesting stuff: "The way they help someone like Jenn, who presents so many unique challenges and doesn't follow the rulebook in treatment, is amazing." These observations made a lasting impression on Amy and would inspire her academic pursuits in the coming years.

Amy also found comfort in the other kids around the rehab center who were facing the similar situation of having a family member with a brain injury. It was late summer when we arrived in Milford, a time when all the young people came daily for visits.

Two young boys, Sidney and Marcus, became especially close friends. The two brothers told Amy the story of how earlier in the summer they were riding with their mom in the family car behind their dad, who was on a motorcycle. They saw him enter an intersection and get hit by an oncoming car. When a motorcycle and a car collide, the outcome for the motorcycle driver is never good, and that was the case with their dad—he was alive but had to be rushed to the hospital in critical condition. Like Jenn, he had suffered a traumatic brain injury. The boys shared details about how dealing with this tragedy had planted vivid images in their minds. Their world was turned upside down just like Amy's, and how their future would unfold was unclear. Would their dad ever be the same? Would he be returning home anytime soon?

Those hot August days at Hillcrest were the best that summer had to offer for Amy, Sidney, and Marcus. Instead of hospital rooms and treatment centers, these friends could play outside or swim in the small pool of the motel next door that was available for Hillcrest families. This offered a much-needed break from the serious nature of all the indoor confinement they had experienced in prior weeks.

The Hillcrest facility was small, but it specialized in rehabilitating people who had sustained a traumatic brain injury. I had no idea how a brain injury presented itself in a patient, and it seemed unimaginable that this was the population that Jennifer now fit into.

Her injury did not look the way it's scripted in Hollywood movies where a person wakes up after a blow to the head and is completely alert, their only repercussion being amnesia. Then a short time later, past memories become vividly clear, and the patient miraculously has a full recovery. Great stuff for a film, but it's not the way a head injury works. For me, this was the only reference I had about what to expect for my Jennifer.

Starved for information on traumatic brain injuries, all the families who had a loved one at the facility were receptive to a special program provided by Hillcrest: lectures on head injury offered on weekends followed by a free luncheon for all to share. It gave families valuable information and brought us together in one location, giving us ample opportunity to talk with each other and share our concerns and fears.

"My son is up and walking but seems off cognitively," a mother told me. I had seen him in the hallways, and I knew she was right.

"Where do you see all of this going?" asked a fellow family member. "I wonder if any clients ever return to a normal life."

If only I knew. All of us wondered how life would look in the coming months or years. None of us had the answer, but just sharing that concern helped us carry the burden that was heavily weighing us down. "Great question," I offered. "I wish I had an answer."

All of us were new to this thing called head injury. We were scared and ill-prepared for the process that was to be our future and had no idea what outcomes to expect. These families were my lifeline and support group. For Amy, the kids who came on those weekends were the best possible distraction and outlet for her feelings and to help her transition from a girl in the middle of a family catastrophe to a strong and resourceful human being.

WHEN FALL CAME, and it was time for our thirteen-year-old Amy to return to school, she told us that she felt different. Trying to fit in with peers who couldn't relate to the burden she was carrying was uncomfortable for her. Other kids didn't understand why she wasn't into all the usual school-day antics, which now seemed silly and trivial to her. "I can't believe the only things my friends think and talk about are who's in their class, who wears makeup now, and what we should be allowed to wear to school."

As a middle schooler, worrying about such things didn't

take on the same significance to her as in prior years. I admired Amy's herculean strength when she walked into the school building that first day in September and tried to act like a normal teenager, talking to friends, chatting about new clothes and music. But almost immediately after starting the school year, she met Ally, a girl whose mother was dying of cancer. Both girls had found somebody who understood the other's struggles.

I could see why Ally and Amy became fast friends. They shared a common thread of pain, suffering, and the feeling of disconnection from so many of their classmates.

A most fortunate outcome of their meeting was that Amy was there for Ally when the time came for her to say goodbye to her mom. She was there to help her friend get through the painful visitation hours and funeral, so much for so young a person to deal with. Once all the traditional ceremonies were completed, they then had each other to help figure out how to move forward with everyday life.

MARK AND AMY shared a common facade of composure; both seemed to be internalizing their grief, probably to protect me. I never saw Amy cry and had only seen Mark teary-eyed a couple of times throughout the early days of the ordeal. Both went to work or school with their feelings of hurt and anguish carefully concealed beneath a mask of normalcy. Mark had no choice but to continue with work to support our family, and Amy had to return to school, as life could not be put on hold waiting for her sister to get better. I could sense that she wanted to present us with no more problems or worries than we already had and would reassure us that everything was just fine with her.

But our family was far from normal. We were no longer four people living under one roof; one of us was an hour's ride away. Our time and focus were on Jenn's rehabilitation, not mundane things like what's for dinner, food shopping, doing laundry, or recreation. We moved in harmony throughout the crisis, but I think that inwardly we were each suffering alone. Reluctant to burden the others with our own emotional upheaval at any particular moment in time, we each did the tasks that were required of us. I didn't know if Mark or Amy fell apart like I did when I was alone. Whenever I had time to myself, I cried. Before falling asleep at night, or when driving home from Jenn's, my tears came freely and many times uncontrollably.

When fall arrived and Amy's soccer season began, Mark would spend the day with Jenn at Hillcrest on weekends while I went with Amy to games and tournaments. Mark and Jenn had always been close and loved to go on little outings together throughout the years before the accident. Now, those outings began again, and took on the form of him pushing Jenn in her wheelchair up and down the streets of Milford so she could enjoy fresh air and new scenery. When Jenn was in a semiconscious state, movement of the wheelchair seemed to be a soothing force. Her body would relax from its constant random movements and a peacefulness came over her; the bumpier the ride, the calmer Jenn was.

With her being more alert as time went on, these outings from the facility took on a different twist. Hillcrest had a new recreation center downtown. Mark would wheel Jenn the few blocks down the street to the building where they had access to the fun equipment inside: air hockey, pin ball machines, an arcade basketball game, and several video game machines. It was here that he made a fascinating discovery: Jenn could play Pac-Man. She couldn't remember how to eat, talk, or walk, but she seemed to remember this video game. The injury had affected some parts of her brain profoundly, while other parts remained intact. Figuring out which parts were damaged and which were unscathed would be our challenge for years to come.

When visiting Jennifer as a family, we often had dinners at the local Pizza House just down the street from Hillcrest. We always brought Jenn with us for these dinners, even though for many months she ate nothing and just sat quietly staring off into space. The owners were always very welcoming and gracious. "Hi, Rubins, come on in, we have a seat for you right over here." And they always acknowledged Jenn, not ignoring her as some people tended to do when we brought her out in public. "Jenn, nice to see you, welcome to the Pizza House." Once we were seated, they would come to our table and ask, "What can we get for you tonight? Will Jenn be having anything? We can't wait for the day when she comes in here and orders salad and pizza. It will happen, we're sure of it."

They spoke more confidently and reassuringly than they may have felt, but it certainly made us feel good and very welcomed in their cozy restaurant.

Months went by with this routine of dinners at the pizza parlor, always with Jenn watching us and not eating. But all Lori's diligent work paid off, and Jenn had finally relearned how to eat. She was tolerant of different tastes and textures, and her table manners had improved remarkably, which made it easier for her to eat in public.

At last, that long-awaited time when Jenn could join us for a pizza had come. "We have your usual table all ready for you," the owner, Mary, said as she escorted us to our seats.

"Bring a place setting for Jenn too. She will be having dinner tonight," Mark said with a proud grin. All of us knew what a big occasion this was.

Mary looked shocked and called to her husband, "Marco, did you hear that? Jenn's going to eat tonight!" Marco came out from the kitchen, excitement written all over his face as he rushed up to us and gave big hugs of congratulations to everyone. "Jenn's dinner is on us," he announced. "She can have anything she wants."

All of Jenn's dinners in the future would be free. They'd never let us pay for her meals. Mary and Marco relished watching her consume food and would give her anything and everything on the menu. These were the first of many people on the long journey ahead of us whose hearts Jenn would deeply touch.

THROUGHOUT THE unfolding months, Mark, Amy, and I watched Jenn's therapy sessions and learned much from them. We were observers, watching her progress, or in some areas, the lack of it. We began seeing how people accepted and interacted with our daughter, although she was unable to verbally respond to them. As Jenn roamed the hallways, she stopped to squeeze people's arms and offer them a smile. Visitors talked to her, and she laughed and had the appearance of understanding them. She gave a wave to anyone who walked past her and patrolled the hallways looking for new faces and curious things to touch and explore. She was known by everyone who worked there or came to visit the facility as the friendly girl who always had an endearing smile on her face.

During that first year and a half, all of us were slowly recovering. Jenn's progress was documented by video tapes from her sessions as well as in written reports. The strides she made over those months were remarkable and evident for all to see. Although not as obvious, Mark, Amy, and I were also healing. Our progress couldn't be measured on charts or graphs; rather, it came in our ability to smile, feel happy, and adjust to the new normal that was now our family.

Chapter 3

WHERE DO WE
GO FROM HERE?

Nineteen months after Jenn first arrived at the Milford rehab center, it was time to relocate her for the next level of care. Given the severity of her injury, Jenn's progress was medically remarkable, but she was far from who she had been before the accident, the way we wished to recapture her. Yes, there were improvements: She now could eat and drink, and she was mobile, walking despite the noticeable limp. But communication was still nonexistent, and there were more missing pieces when comparing the original version of my daughter to the one who now appeared before me. It was hard to find Jenn's original personality and demeanor—she'd always been dignified and statuesque, but all those signature characteristics were gone. It was hard to comprehend the extent of what had happened to her and figure out how I could get my original daughter back.

At seventeen, Jennifer had been a striking blonde with a calm, gentle manner. She captured everyone's eye as she entered a room with a quiet energy and an air of sophistication that was quite mesmerizing and glamorous. A good student, she excelled in the sciences like her father, a physics and earth science teacher. Although she participated in various sports throughout her school years, she didn't have a true competitive nature and was never a standout on the soccer field or tennis court. Skiing was her specialty—not as a competitor, but more like a graceful dancer as she glided down the mountain terrain in rhythmic serpentine curves of measured precision and elegance.

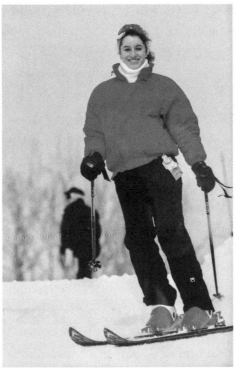

Jenn skiing pre-accident.

NEAT TO A FAULT, Jenn's room was always the most organized area of our home. Drawers were carefully arranged, with even the smallest items located in just the right place to keep all sections in perfect order.

Jenn and Amy didn't look like sisters, and the two girls had entirely different personalities. Jenn was the taller, soft-spoken, and graceful one; Amy was small in stature but had a big, bubbly personality willing to take on the world with energy and determination.

Very social and with a core group of friends, Jenn had been happy and on top of the world. The summer of the accident, she was looking forward to her senior year in high school. She had been working part time as a cashier in the local hardware store, which provided spending money to put gas in the car and for entertainment. With a driver's license and cash in hand, Jenn had the sense of freedom all teenagers love. This mobile freedom was an especially fun way for her to take her younger sister out for ice cream or a movie. For siblings, their relationship was easy, pleasant, and presented few conflicts. Both girls had their own separate interests and friends, and they could just enjoy time together.

Dinner at our house often included at least one of Amy or Jennifer's friends. Always welcomed into our home, friends added to the conversations and no topics were off-limits. We didn't experience teenage rebellion from either Jenn or Amy. All members of our family were treated with respect and dignity, and we all truly enjoyed each other's company.

The new Jennifer, who was finally able to walk the halls of Hillcrest unattended, had little resemblance to the girl I'd raised for the past seventeen years. More like a bull in a china shop, she again drew everyone's eye as she entered a room, but not for the same reasons. No longer was she a graceful glow of perfection—she was loud and inappropriate. Her calm and gentle nature was replaced with an anxious, frustrated, and excitable one. Early on, a neuropsychologist told me that Jenn's injury would leave her with many holes in her basic personality. At that point in time, it was hard for me to see any of the original Jenn. The holes were cavernous, and I despaired when I saw all the parts that were missing.

After careful research, facilitated by the Brain Injury Association of New York State, we decided to relocate Jenn to the Datahr facility in Brookfield, Connecticut, an hour's drive from our home in Washingtonville. When she arrived at Datahr in March of 1993, she was starting the next chapter in her post-accident life. Within the Datahr organization, we thought their group home on Squire Court would serve well as Jenn's new residence. Here she would continue to receive her basic rehab services of physical and occupational therapy as well as speech, but in a less institutional setting. The group home also provided support services for her daily living needs such as personal hygiene and meals.

On a quiet, upscale, residential street, this group home was a barn-red, single-story house with white trim and a semicircular driveway in front for staff and visitor parking. The flat walkway leading up to the front door was perfect for Jenn to navigate without concern for her tripping on steps or uneven surfaces.

Upon entering the home, my attention was directed to the five staff members who gathered to greet us in the living room area just beyond the wide-open foyer. Dressed casually in jeans and T-shirts, the two young men and three women were a striking difference from the uniformed nursing staff that had been a part of Jenn's post-accident life up to this

point. Each stepped forward to shake our hand and introduce themselves with warm, friendly smiles.

But with the smell of fresh-baked chocolate chip cookies
in the air, Jenn's attention was immediately drawn to the
kitchen just off to the left. That tantalizing scent kicked Jenn
into high gear. Screaming her happy noise, she charged in
and immediately headed to the kitchen to snatch up as many
of the cookies as she could get her hands on. Fortunately,
she was only able to grab a few before staff made quick work
of securing the remaining ones in a cabinet.

That was Jenn's grand entrance into what was to be her
new home. The sound of her voice of happiness when she
caught a whiff of those cookies was the brash introduction to
what staff could expect from their new charge. Inappropriately
loud and shrill, the sound she made grated like nails on a
blackboard. Though no one wanted to deny her that moment
of total joy she was expressing, it was hard to listen to. It was
unlike any sound Jenn had made before her accident. Perhaps
there was some damage in her vocal cords that presented
itself when she pressed them to their extreme limits with her
overexcited vocalization. Whatever the case, her noises were
quite a challenge, even painful, for those around her.

The staff, who looked notably alarmed, did their best
to welcome Jenn and our family, but I knew they had to
be wondering how this new client would possibly fit in to
their home and how it would work to have her live there.
They'd been briefed on Jenn's injuries, so they were aware
of some of the challenges to be faced, but having her charge
in with such a loud and aggressive manner seemed to really
put them on notice. I knew Jenn was unlike anyone they
had ever worked with due to her lack of communication.
No one we had encountered since her accident, even in

the professional world of rehab and brain injury, had ever worked with a client like her. Immediately they started asking questions that hadn't been addressed in their briefing. "How will we know what she wants or needs?"

"Was it easy to tell that she wanted those cookies?" I asked. "Many of her signals are very obvious; others are subtle, and I'll help you learn how to read them."

"Is she violent?" asked the young man named Joe.

"Not really. She did some biting in the past but has outgrown that phase. She just gets vocally loud when she is mad."

"How do we communicate with her and teach her daily skills?" asked the blonde woman who introduced herself as Chris.

"That's more complicated, and again, I'll be here to help you learn the techniques that have been employed up to this point." I loved their eagerness to ask and learn about Jenn, and I knew that given time, they would figure it out, just as the rest of us had.

These were valid concerns for the staff awaiting us that first day. Jenn's integration into a new environment meant that I would be going every day to the facility to be with her and work with staff. Fortunately, they quickly grasped the idea that they should talk to Jenn just as they would any other person. Their body language would help bridge the gap between words she didn't understand, and she could be guided to carry on with daily routines as if she comprehended some of what they said to her. Just as we would talk with a small child to get them to mimic things we want them to do before they learn to speak, staff, family, and friends would have to do the same with Jenn.

For her part, when Jenn wanted to get someone's attention, she knew to make eye contact. If her noises didn't have you looking at her, she would grab your hand, squeeze your arm, or, if that didn't work, she would put her face directly in front of yours. Once she'd made eye contact, she would direct you to what she wanted with a shift of her eyes to the thing she was interested in, such as a sandwich or someone else's food. She would also physically take you to where she wanted to go by grasping your hand and leading you to places like the refrigerator, the kitchen table, or her bedroom.

In addition to making noises and eye contact, Jenn employed engaging facial expressions to convey her wants and needs. Her big smile and the twinkle in her eye gave you all the information you needed to understand when she was happy and excited. And there was never a doubt when she was unhappy or angry. Loud vocal protests, along with the grimace of her mouth and brows that came together in an expression of serious dismay, let us know that she wanted no part of what was being asked of her. Everyone hoped that one day, all the dots would connect in her brain, and she would understand what we were saying. Until then, we continued our one-way conversations with her that must have appeared very normal to outside observers.

BEFORE BRINGING JENN to Datahr, we had toured the main facility where the corporate offices and therapy rooms were located and carefully looked at the residence where she would live. Datahr's group home on Squire Court was very well thought-out and neatly maintained. There was little question in our minds this was the perfect place-ment for our daughter. It felt like a true family home, not institutional in any way. The living room had a double set of sliding doors that opened to the patio and backyard. The two walls on either side of the sliding doors had built-in bookcases tastefully trimmed to match the white molding running throughout the interior. On the wall opposite the bookcases was another built-in cabinet housing the large TV that could be easily viewed from either of the two couches placed at a right angle to each other or the armchair that graced the corner. Equally impressive were the Ethan Allen furnishings throughout the house, all carefully chosen and arranged by one of that company's interior decorators. This home had a real "wow" factor for Mark, Amy, and me.

Beyond the main living area, there were two wings each with three bedrooms, a large, shared bathroom, and a sitting area complete with a sofa, comfy armchair, and television. This specially designed residence was perfect for six clients to have their private spaces, but still offer all the comforts of any family home.

I would soon learn the reason for the high-quality furnishings that so complemented Squire's living space. The Ethan Allen headquarters was located in the neighboring town of Danbury. It was their expertise and generosity that helped Datahr give this relatively new group home the welcoming appearance and elegance that made me feel good about where my daughter was going to live.

WITH A WORK schedule to keep, Mark was only able to visit Jenn in Connecticut on weekends, while I stayed with Amy to attend her soccer events. Over the past year, we had learned that Jenn loved riding in the car, so Mark would drive her around the countryside and through local towns, sharing time and one-sided conversations with her. He started doing this the first weekend after we brought her to Squire and continued the same routine for many months. He told me she was a quiet passenger, content to just look out the window and be with her dad. They would always make a lunch stop along the way, and when the weather turned nice, they occasionally tried to walk the sidewalks of an interesting residential area Mark might find.

After spending the day with Jenn, Mark always wanted to share with me how their time together had gone. Week after week, he would report that Jenn was happy as long as he was driving, and she certainly liked their lunch stops, but the walking part always presented a problem. Jenn wasn't one to appreciate walking without a purpose.

After one particular visit, Mark's frustration boiled over as he described how he tried to walk with her on a residential street in New Milford, a neighboring town to Brookfield. Mark said she would turn into any walkway leading to a house and when he redirected her away from the residence she would have a raging fit. "Man, she put up such a fuss, I was afraid someone would call the police thinking I was hurting her."

He went on with his story, "I had to physically push her away from the entrance of each house, until she spotted the next house and thought that was our destination. She would start running up to that walkway until I stopped her. Once again, she'd start yelling and try to push past me to get to the door." On and on it went as Mark tried unsuccessfully to navigate the street with her.

After a couple attempts to walk in residential neighborhoods with Jenn, Mark gave it up. Instead, he located some local walking trails, thinking that here she wouldn't target doorways as her destination and wouldn't become so frustrated. And he wouldn't be at risk of someone calling the police on him.

WHEN OUR GIRLS were young, Mark enjoyed baking with them, and apple pies were their favorite thing to make. There were no shortcuts in the process, which meant making the crust from scratch. I quickly learned that it was best for me to vacate the kitchen, as these three had their own way of doing things. It didn't necessarily follow the format I would have used—they'd peel apples with the wrong knife, use too much flour to roll out the dough, use a fork where I thought they should use a knife, and would use a spoon when a spatula would have been the better tool. But once they were finished, the pie was delicious, the kitchen was clean, and the girls had experienced hours of fun in the kitchen with their dad.

In our family, tradition has it that sometimes what seems like a disaster at the time can turn into a funny story remembered and repeated for years to come. One particular pie holds the honor of such a story. When the girls were about six and ten years old, after making their amazing and perfect apple pie, Mark and the girls set it on the worktable in the garage to cool in the fall air. They didn't think too much of it when our Siamese cat, Cookie, followed them into the garage. Just as they set the pie down, Cookie decided to leap up on the table to see what was going on—and ended up right in the middle of their culinary creation. The perfect pie now had two holes going into the center where Cookie's front feet had landed. We couldn't really blame the cat—she didn't know the pie was there—and like us, she wasn't too happy about what happened. After I gave her a quick rinse in the mud sink, Cookie was left to finish the grooming process and clean any remaining yucky sweet mess from her legs and especially from between her toes.

But what should we do about all that hard work and the perfect pie? Well, truth be told, we ate it anyway. We carefully scooped out the area immediately around the leg holes and consumed the rest. Lesson learned: make sure no cats are in the garage when pies are cooling.

After Jenn's accident, Mark wanted to recapture the pleasure he'd had baking with the girls. Apple pies were a bit too challenging under the new circumstances, but cupcakes seemed a good substitute, with less arduous directions for Jenn to follow. Together they made lots of batches of cupcakes at Squire, with Jenn doing many of the tasks like cracking the eggs, mixing the ingredients, and scooping batter into each of the waiting cupcake papers.

Just as Jenn remembered how to play Pac-Man, she remembered how to crack eggs. This was an especially fun part for her in making the cupcakes. Years before when she was a child, dad had shown her his one-handed technique of cracking eggs and pulling them apart. It was an old memory that came to the surface, and one that Jenn could do flawlessly.

Once the cupcakes were baked and set out to cool, it was hard for Jenn to wait before eating them. Mark learned it was best to take a drive with her and then return a short time later to add the frosting. Upon their return to Squire, he showed Jenn how to scoop out the colorful premade icing from its plastic container and cover the top of each cupcake. Finally, it was time for Jenn's favorite part of the process—eating. She would devour her share in seconds.

THE HARDEST PART of any visit for both Mark and me was saying goodbye to Jenn when it was time for us to head home. She would become notably upset when she saw we were walking out the door without her. Tears were often shed as she clung to our arm or tried to follow us outside. It ripped our hearts out to leave her behind, but we couldn't stay indefinitely, and we couldn't always bring her home with us. We couldn't provide the continuing care she required, and this was the best place for her to be, but that didn't make it any easier. As often as not, I too came to tears as I headed to the car and left my precious daughter behind, looking through the side windows of the doorway and watching me as I moved beyond her line of vision and disappeared to wherever she thought I was going.

In time, we found that if a staff member took Jenn off for a ride before we left, she was much happier. But the sad look on her face, even as they pulled away or when we left her standing at the group home, still haunts us. Everyone assured us that once we were gone, Jenn quickly returned to her happy self and continued with her day or evening. "You know that she's fine once you are gone and she can't see you any longer, right?" the staff assured us. Her drama lasted only the few minutes it took for us to walk out the door and down the driveway, but that still didn't make it less heart-wrenching. I sometimes felt that if I could have explained to her why she needed to stay and have her understand, it would have been easier. But I doubted even that would have helped my overwhelming grief. I hated leaving her; every time, it was beyond unbearable as we slowly made our way to the car. Mark and I both felt we were turning our back on her, abandoning her, when all we really wanted to do was embrace her and make all our suffering disappear. It didn't matter that we might be returning the very next day. It didn't help that we had just seen her the day before. The parting was always painful, each and every time, like a self-inflicted torture that we had to endure for eternity.

Chapter 4

THE LAWSUIT

During Jenn's rehabilitation and relocation, the lawsuits against the drivers involved in her accident continued to progress, and a trial date was finally set. It had taken almost three years from the date of the accident to reach this point.

Having worked in a law office, I knew that even if a person or company had insurance coverage, the money would not automatically be paid out, even when liability is evident—money only changes hands when lawsuits are filed and won. The accident report left no question about who was at fault, but the battle had to be handled in a court of law. The stakes were high, both in terms of Jenn's needs and the dollar amount held by the insurance companies under their clients' policies. This was to be the first of a continuing lesson for me that the job of an insurance company was to keep their money. My job was to get it from them to help Jenn.

As the court date neared, I became more anxious about the idea of facing the driver of the cement truck.

Still distraught to put a face on the person I learned was a woman, I was deeply unsettled about seeing her in person. I was willing to come before the court blindfolded or make an appearance only when she would not be present. Our attorneys were vague on how that would work and how the court would respond to my request, but I was adamant about the need for her visual identity not to be revealed to me. I couldn't bear seeing this person's face in the local mall or grocery. If I didn't know what she looked like, I could freely patronize local businesses without any fear of knowing she might be there at the same time.

With jury selection completed, Mark and I arrived at the courthouse on the first day of the trial, prepared for the emotional and disturbing ordeal that was expected to take place. As we walked up the steps of the courthouse in Goshen, New York, on that sunny day in June, we knew this was not going to be pleasant, but we were anxious to have it all behind us.

Our legal team was prepared to exhibit photographs of the vehicles and accident site, something we had not wanted to see. Details of the accident investigation would be gone over in explicit detail, as would the extent of Jenn's injuries. Jenn's medical charts would be reviewed for the jury, and graphic documents would be carefully laid out for them to understand the extent of her suffering and the consequences leading to her disabilities. Film footage from Hillcrest was going to be shared as well as footage of her from before the accident.

Gathered around the foyer outside of the courtroom, attorneys from the opposing sides clustered in their respective groups, strategizing and conferring by phone with their clients. Several lawyers were there representing the driver, Rachael, whose car Jenn had been in. The company that employed the truck driver at the time of the accident also had legal representation. I was careful not to look in that direction, as I was afraid of being able to pick out the driver from the group. I didn't know whether she was there or not. Everyone was dressed in business attire, making it harder to tell attorneys from defendants. Finally, there were four lawyers working on our team: Marc, our attorney, the two other partners from his law firm, plus Steve, a trial attorney brought in to present our case to the jury.

Our legal counselors were closely gathered around Mark and me as we waited to be ushered into the courtroom.

"I know this is going to be emotionally hard for the two of you," Steve began, "but we have a solid case. It's just a matter of getting all the insurance money available. They're going to try and get us to settle for a smaller amount, but that isn't going to happen. I'm going to push for the whole thing."

No sooner were the words out of his mouth than he was approached by an attorney from the opposing side. Negotiations had begun. Still outside the courtroom, all the attorneys seemed to be scrambling, first talking to one set of lawyers and then moving on to the next. I hadn't expected this kind of informal haggling outside the courtroom. It was all done in hushed voices. Conversations were whispered as watchful eyes made sure no one was close enough to hear what was being discussed. When attorneys approached our group, they would very quietly ask if they could have a word with Steve. They would walk a short distance away with him to have their conversation before he returned to our circle and told us the latest offerings.

After about twenty minutes of this flurry of activity, the judge called for representatives from each side to meet with him separately in his private chambers. For the next round he called all the opposing sides in at the same time.

In the midst of the negotiations, Steve reported back to us, "The judge is pushing all sides to come to an agreement to avoid the long trial that's headed our way. But so far, the insurance company is only offering seventy-five percent of their holdings, so we have no deal." Mark and I were relieved that Steve held his position because, like him, we wanted all the insurance money available. Jenn would need it, and that was what that insurance money was for.

Our legal team was unwavering in their determination to win the entire sum of insurance money available. Each time they were called in, they stubbornly held their position. It became clear to the defense teams that our side was more than willing to bring our case before the jury. As Steve would tell us later, after what he felt was endless ridiculous haggling, he made his position clear: "We want it all, or we'll see you in trial, period!"

He was not going to accept anything less than the entire sum of the insurance claim. Fear finally prevailed as the insurance companies seemed to anticipate that an even larger settlement might be awarded by a jury, thus exposing their client to a financial judgment against their business. They relented on the first day of trial, before we even entered the courtroom. At last, three long years after the lawsuit was filed, it was finally settled. Relief washed over us like a tsunami. We walked away victorious—the feeling was euphoric.

IN THE MONTHS leading up to the court date, our lawyers were working to understand and prepare documents needed for Jenn to qualify for a new kind of trust made available in the legal system. With this new trust structure, the settlement would be protected for the true benefit of the recipient. Prior to 1991, all monies collected from a lawsuit went directly to the recipient. Jenn's case would be the first in New York State to allow the money to be put in a supplemental needs trust.

This unique financial instrument had a significant effect on how we were able to rebuild a life for her that would be both meaningful and fulfilling. It allowed us to use Medicaid to pay for her basic care, which was a huge benefit in a facility that cost many tens of thousands of dollars each year. With the basics taken care of, the trust was then available for all the extra expenses that made a life worth living. As bad as it sounded for the Medicaid system, it really wasn't. The amount of Jenn's settlement was enough to generate sufficient income and growth to maintain the principal, even as it covered all the costly extras we provided for her. Without the trust, the money would have been quickly drained down and gone in a few years just paying for her daily housing and care expenses at Datahr. At that point, Jenn would have had no money and ended up on Medicaid, which would have held her back from the many enriching experiences that the trust could provide for her.

"Make sure this money makes a difference in Jennifer's life." This was the parting statement our lawyers gave us after years of legal battling to get us that settlement. Easy for them to say but what exactly was it that would make this "difference"?

After much thought and soul-searching about this challenge, our family determined the following things were necessary: a car for mobility, ready cash for daily expenditures, a personal attendant to take Jenn places and do things with her, and training of staff so they understood our goals and expectations and how to attain them. We also needed the facility to be willing to go along with our unprecedented guide-lines and allow me to work side by side with the employees who would serve as Jenn's personal attendants.

Little did I know the story that would unfold: My daughter, despite her extreme disabilities, would affect so many lives in a positive way. She would make a lasting impression on her caregivers and would be forever cemented into the fabric of their families.

Chapter 5

A NEW PHASE

Five months after arriving at Datahr, the lawsuit was settled, and it was time for me to begin hiring the personal staff who would be working with Jenn.

I kept an eye out for potential candidates among the many Datahr employees I saw while visiting each day, so I had a head start in the hiring process. I wanted young women similar in age to Jenn, who would have the appearance of being her peers. I thought it was important for Jenn to feel that she had friends she did things with, not just assistants who took care of her basic needs. These women had to be trustworthy, willing to try new things, and have the kind of energy that would translate into being a fun companion for my daughter.

Datahr posted the positions for personal attendants and the screening process began. I wasn't surprised that there were few applicants.

"Barb, you know that many people are reluctant to commit to working with a client they viewed as extremely challenging to manage," Squire staff pointed out to me. Jenn's reputation was known throughout the agency.

Despite this hurdle, I was able to gradually fill all the positions in a rather short time. Some hires quickly fell by the wayside. They were dedicated and kind but really didn't have the creative touch to move beyond basic homecare.

This was all new territory for me: figuring out what Jenn's days would look like and how to make it all come together. I plowed ahead and tried to give the impression I was one hundred percent sure of what I was doing. But inside, I was not the self-assured person I was projecting for the world to see. I didn't know what would work and what would be a total disaster as I trained my new hires and developed the treatment programs I wanted them to use with Jenn. I knew I was the one who could make Jenn's life better and more complete. Mark had work and couldn't devote the time needed to oversee all of this. Sure, there were professionals around, but none had the vested interest in Jenn that I did.

Doubts plagued me about what I was creating for her, but I only shared those feelings with Mark. He was my safe sounding board. I could brainstorm with him about my ideas and concerns without revealing my uncertainties to the people in Connecticut.

"Mark, I can't imagine all the things I need to show the new people and the best way to go about it. I don't even know what I want them to do with her. We haven't done much in the way of new and interesting activities with Jenn since her accident. So, what I'm asking them to do are things we haven't even done."

"Just give yourself time to work with them and see how things go," he reassured me. "We don't know what can or cannot be done with Jenn, but this is the way we find out. I think everything will become clearer once you start exploring options with the new people, try different things with them, and see how Jenn responds."

I could always count on Mark to be encouraging and supportive. Without him I would have been hopelessly lost.

ALL THE LOGISTICS of having a car for Jenn were ironed out between the trust and the legal team at Datahr. It was a complicated process, and many organizations would have balked at all the red tape involved and simply denied my plan. Not so with Datahr—they were on board and very supportive to help me implement my idea of having a private car for Jenn's use and insuring it along with their fleet of vehicles.

All was in place for me to start the Jenn-specific training with my new hires. Armed with all the standard guidelines and procedures for caregiving that came with being a Datahr employee, the one-on-ones still needed to be taught the unique personalized care that I expected from them.

First and foremost, Jenn's safety had to be addressed both in the group home and—even more importantly—when taking her out in public. This concern would prove to be an ongoing issue that needed continued tweaking as new and unexpected situations arose.

I also needed to convey to my staff the extreme nervousness that Mark and I felt about Jenn riding in a car. Our fears were well founded; we knew what a crash did to families. Repeated nightmares of cars colliding plagued me from the dark shadows of my mind. The sound of glass shattering and the squeal of tires were immediately followed by panicked voices from one of my loved ones. I tried to call out to them from the wreckage, but words didn't reach my lips. I struggled and fought my way to shout the word that kept evading me. *Help!* In my desperation to yell, I would finally awaken myself from the horrific scene.

It was my deep-seated fear of cars that I had to convey to the staff and the staff had to understand where I was coming from with my concerns. Getting our staff to drive safely proved to be the easy part to implement; it was all the *other stuff* that presented the greatest challenges.

Helping my young staff to anticipate dangerous situations for Jenn took time. There were no specific things I could tell them to watch out for or be careful of—that kind of understanding would only come from them experiencing Jenn's daily routine and discovering potential hazards. It wasn't just the sharp, hot, or poison things I was worried about; it was also the mischief Jenn could get up to if unmonitored.

When Jenn resided at Hillcrest, I had learned the kind of antics she could get into. In the mornings before I came or in the late afternoons after I left, she could freely roam on her own. With total mobility, she wandered the halls with the curiosity of a toddler trying to learn about her surroundings. She wanted to touch, taste, and collect things.

The first collection happened early one morning before I arrived. As soon as I stepped off the elevator, three nurses joined me and laughingly shared Jenn's latest escapade. During their routine of getting clients ready for the day ahead, they noticed all the toothbrushes were missing.

Jenn was still in a wheelchair at this time but had no trouble getting herself around the facility. They discovered later that Jenn had gone into each room, grabbed the toothbrushes, and once she had them all, deposited them in her trash can.

Everyone understood that Jenn hated having her teeth brushed, and three people were needed to perform this task: one to restrain her arms and hands, another to keep her mouth wedged open with a tongue depressor, and the third person to do the actual brushing. It was easy for me to imagine why Jenn decided to take matters into her own hands—no toothbrushes, no brushing.

This caper generated a lot of laughs around Hillcrest and showed a cleverness and resourcefulness on Jenn's part that hadn't been seen since before her accident, and this became a favorite, fun story to talk about. Jennifer's new quirky personality was starting to present itself. People began seeing her and many of her actions as humorous—a big change in how she was perceived. We had all tended to define her as severely disabled, a sad case of TBI with few positives attached to it. For people to see her in this new light was refreshing but strange to me.

Her collections continued, but the one that was troubling to the staff was when Jenn took the portable urinals that hung on the male clients' wheelchairs. It was a mystery: why urinals? That was the final straw. The administrators decided Jenn needed to have personal staff whose sole job was watching her throughout the day when I wasn't there. Staff members specifically dedicated to Jenn were even more necessary when she started walking, as she now had access to items that she couldn't reach when in a wheelchair. The expense for that coverage had been included as part of the facility's basic charge for her care at Hillcrest but not at Datahr.

At Squire, the staff kept an eye on all the clients, but I knew Jenn would get into a lot of trouble without someone specifically assigned to watch her every move. That's why I was there every day to monitor her and keep her entertained. Once

Jenn's new staff members were on board, my job was to train them to be on the alert for anything that would endanger Jenn or the things around her, such as equipment or furnishings.

Jenn kept herself busy with kitchen raids and rearranging or hiding things all day and sometimes at night. Her staff had to continuously keep an eye on her. But she seemed to be keenly aware that people were monitoring her, and when they were distracted, she'd sneak a snack from the kitchen or hide something she may have thought was out of place.

An unsupervised kitchen trashcan offered an endless variety of treats for Jenn's obsessive hunger. She must have made a mental note when someone threw leftovers in the trash. She kept watch, and when no one was looking, in a flash she'd grab the food and stuff it quickly into her mouth. All of us caught her at this trick. Sometimes she stuffed so much in at once that she looked like a chipmunk. She'd quickly chew and swallow before someone told her to spit the food out.

Leg and hand braces would often disappear, later to be found in the bottom of the garbage. Jenn learned that if she placed them on top, they'd quickly be found. Devices or equipment that Jenn perceived as being in her way would be tossed across the room or brushed onto the floor. She would rearrange papers left on a table, pick decals off equipment, and take remotes from electronic devices and hide them under a furniture cushion. And she rummaged through unattended purses looking for tasty treats inside.

She took car keys that staff left on a table or counter and put them away—her kind of away—in a drawer, the trash, or under a sofa cushion. Was she trying to keep everyone in the house after their shift was over, or was she just cleaning up? We never knew. Jenn was always on the move, and hiding keys was only one of her many daily activities.

AN ESSENTIAL PART of my training focused on how to direct Jenn to comply with our directions with the least amount of resistance. It was necessary for her staff to have creative tools to manage her behaviors. I needed to train them on how to do some very basic things: come with me, walk, sit, and wait. Well, waiting was still a problem!

The staff learned how to communicate with Jenn by mimicking me.

I got Jenn's attention by saying her name. Once she looked at me, I'd use hand signals and point to what I wanted her to do. "Jenn, let's go," I motioned for her to come. This usually worked fine, especially if I pointed at the front door or showed her the car keys.

To get Jenn up and go with me, if I was not pointing to the kitchen or front door and had no keys in my hand, most often it took offering my hands to help pull her up. "Come on Jenn, time to get up." Resistance to standing up usually only happened in a restaurant or at the kitchen table. She would take my hands for the added oomph to propel herself upright. Did she need this assistance to stand? No. She always giggled as though she'd put one over on me and seemed to enjoy the game.

Getting her to sit required less effort: make eye contact, gesture to the chair, and pat it for her to sit. Easy enough, except that once seated she would most likely pop right back up and be ready to go again. Jenn was wired tightly those first few years with an energy and anxiety that was boundless. Getting her to sit for more than a few minutes didn't happen unless she was eating, riding in a car, or being constantly entertained with an activity. Learning how to get her to sit or stand were just two of the directives for the staff to learn. The list was endless. There were cues for all the various daily routines, and more would be added as needed.

There were many other aspects of the job description for my workers beyond caring for Jenn. The car needed regular maintenance such as tire-pressure checks, oil changes, washes, and appointments for repairs as needed. I wanted staff to take responsibility for caring for this vehicle.

My knowledge of car maintenance hovered around zero. My husband, Mark, always took care of anything associated with our vehicles, so I employed his expertise to set up repair and maintenance guidelines for them to follow with Jenn's car. He wrote a detailed calendar of tasks and carefully researched and listed the best places to get each service done. This was so like Mark, detail oriented and precise in all of his undertakings.

I also expected the staff members to do Jenn's at home physical and occupational therapy programs—PT and OT—each day. As in the past, the OT work on her right arm and hand continued to be challenging. She was particularly uncooperative when the person was a "newbie" who was afraid of hurting her. Jenn resisted allowing them to touch her and would yell to scare them away. It usually worked and was a sign that the staff needed more training and experience. This was where I stepped in and revealed the true nature of Jenn's protests.

"She knows you're new and is just trying to scare you away. What you're doing isn't hurting her; she just doesn't like to be touched or bothered with. We have to do these exercises to maintain her range of motion. Try again, and don't let her pull away; be kind but firm in your approach," I explained. With that Jenn would settle down and allow them to proceed.

Selecting clothing and cosmetics for Jenn was yet another task I needed them to do. They had to learn what I considered tasteful attire and the appropriate price. I wanted Jenn to look nice and resemble my pre-accident daughter who was always stylish and concerned about her appearance.

As the need for clothing arose, one of the staff members, Jenn, and I would go shopping at the local Danbury Fair Mall. She seemed to enjoy picking out clothes from the racks, but it was a challenge getting her to try things on.

"Jenn take off your shirt," I directed while giving her shirt a little tug upward.

Moaning a little, she pulled it off and threw it at me. "Nice throw Jenn. Now put this one on."

After having her put the new shirt on and us checking it out, I now wanted her to remove it. "Take it off, Jenn." Moans of protests were leveled at me. She didn't use her high-volume setting, but her voice echoed throughout the dressing room area.

Trying on pants required removing her shoes and leg brace. I learned that it was better to buy pants and try them on at home when she was getting dressed for the first time in the morning rather than in the store. No one cared if she was loud at home, and it worked better that way for all of us.

At first, I went with the girls when they bought Jenn's clothes. Eventually, they were confident enough to make the selections on their own, and then shopping sprees became a fun girls' adventure. Shopping was a good excuse to check out distant outlets or malls for a full day's outing or even an overnight trip.

A huge part of caring for Jenn was to keep her busy with meaningful activities and entertainment. I didn't want her to spend hours sitting on the sofa watching movies or drifting around the house looking for something to pick apart or destroy. All too often people who were disabled simply got "stored" away with little stimulation rather than experiencing a real life. I wanted staff to find interesting things to do with Jenn, like concerts, sporting events, festivals, and new places to explore that would get her out and involved in the community.

I was preparing for Jenn's future. I wanted her to be involved with as many people as possible and have experiences similar to her peers. I couldn't give her the excitement and adventures I wanted for her. I was still crippled with the loss of my original Jennifer. The new young people I brought into her life were vibrant and fun—which I was not. I thought having a network of people in place who understood that community activities should be an integral part of Jenn's life was paramount for her.

AS PART OF my training program, I required every new staff member to watch films taken of Jenn before her accident and then early clips taken at the Milford facility. Each month at Hillcrest, patients were videotaped during all their therapy sessions, clear documentation of client progress. I used various segments of these clips to compile my training video.

Two of Jenn's caregivers, Chris and Suzanne, would later tell me they were horrified by these early videos of Jenn at Hillcrest. Looking at the images of this girl, slumped in her wheelchair, dazed, and only semi-responsive to stimulation, was heartbreaking.

"Barb, I just can't believe how awful those first videos of Jenn were. I couldn't stop crying as I saw her so out-of-it and dazed," Chris said, "but the PT sessions were interesting, especially when they started to get Jenn walking—that was really neat."

"The OT sessions were hard to watch," Suzanne added. "I actually took the training video home to show my husband, and he got upset and said, 'Why are you showing me this; it's painful, and I can't stand to look at it.'"

I had to agree that the footage of occupational therapy, where work was done to try to regain function of her right hand and arm, was alarming. Jenn's facial expressions and loud moaning spoke volumes about the severity of her injury and the pain she was enduring. By comparison, clips of the outgoing, perky, and confident pre-accident Jenn were both insightful and sad when they recognized how different she was.

"I loved seeing Jenn before the accident. It is amazing to see the soft-spoken person she was," Chris commented.

Suzanne totally disagreed with Chris. "I found it hard to watch the video of her before the accident. It was just too much to imagine what all happened to her—that hurt even more than not knowing who she was before."

I knew it was uncomfortable for anyone to watch the training video I put together, but I needed the new staff to understand the severity of Jenn's TBI and to see how far she had come since her accident. I knew it would pull on their heartstrings just as it had on mine when I witnessed the Hillcrest sessions. Having them see the pre-accident Jennifer revealed the daughter I was trying to recapture. Disabilities from a brain injury mask what the original person was really like. With altered personalities and compromised bodies, people with TBIs can seem light-years away from who they were before their injury.

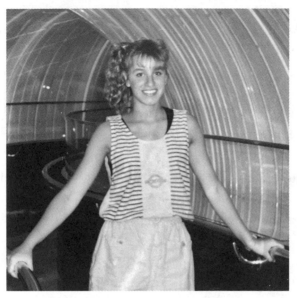

Jenn pre-accident, the girl I was trying to recapture.

For me, it was imperative for Jenn's staff to recognize her as someone who had endured unimaginable hurdles and accomplished a great deal in recovery before coming into their care. Along with understanding would come empathy. I wanted to touch the hearts of her caregivers and give them a reason to go beyond the checklist of required daily tasks in caring for her. The staff needed to be devoted, protective, and a voice for my daughter when faced with situations where she could not fend for herself. Jenn's staff had to fill my shoes when I wasn't there.

FOR MOST OF the next year, I made several trips a week to Brookfield for the training of my staff and to spend time with Jenn. No other client in the facility had a family member who persisted in the oversight of their loved one to this degree. Was this intimidating for staff? I am sure it was, but I didn't

care. Until the time Jenn came to Squire, either Mark or I
had been with her every day since her accident. But after a
few months of daily training sessions with Jenn's private staff,
I began cutting back on my visits. I felt guilty when I wasn't
with her, but it was time to relax my oversight just a bit. I
knew that Jenn was safe, but that didn't make it any easier to
relinquish control to others.

After months of training, the girls were set to handle
things on their own, but I still traveled at least once a week
to Brookfield to check on their progress, spend time with
Jenn, and reevaluate what was going well and what needed
improvement. At any one time, I had three girls who were
responsible for Jenn's care: Two full-time and one part-time
personal staff were required to cover the hours between seven
in the morning and eleven at night, every day of the week.

WHEN WE BROUGHT Jenn to Datahr, Tom Fanning
was the CEO and was still closely connected to some of the
founders of the organization. In 1953, a small group of families
wanted a place where their loved one could have a meaningful
life despite having Down syndrome or some other intellectual
disability. They wanted a safe place for their family member to
be happy and learn new skills. The families originally named
their organization the Danbury Association to Advance the
Handicapped and Retarded. In 1989 they took on the acro-
nym of DATAHR. This name was changed again in 2003 to
Ability Beyond Disability to better reflect the mission of the
organization as a community-based service provider.

As Datahr grew, so did the dreams of the founding families as they structured an organization to give an adult child
an opportunity to be involved in the community and offer a

family style living environment in a group home. Within a few years, they added clients with head injuries to their roster. The needs of that population fit into their model of care.

I don't recall the number of homes they had in their system at the time Jenn arrived on the scene, but I would guess about twenty-six. Squire Court was one that the organization had built using an architectural plan specifically designed for their clients' purposes. Their model was so successful that it was copied and duplicated by agencies in other states.

These founders saw a problem and came up with a solution that served their family members well. They were able to think creatively and create an organization that gave dignity to this population along with opportunities to flourish socially, mentally, and physically. Their facility was just what I needed for our daughter.

Creative thinking was very prevalent when Jenn arrived at Datahr. Tom had seen the positive results that came from families who were determined to build a better life for their child and give them every chance to succeed with as much independence as possible. As CEO, he brought the organization to the highest levels of esteem and consumer outcomes. Datahr, later Ability, became a leader in the industry for the care of individuals with traumatic brain injuries and intellectual disabilities.

It is hard for an organization to break from the norm when they have a tried and tested framework of procedures that are established and working successfully, but Tom was supportive of my training and program ideas and gave me as much leniency as possible. He came to expect that I would test all norms, but he let me know that he understood Jenn was unlike any other client they had served and required a unique tailoring of programs for her care.

Employees do not take clients home, right? This seemed like a logical rule, even if there was nothing in writing stating that fact. Work should have a clear separation from one's personal family life, shouldn't it? That was an industry standard, but it was the exact opposite of what I had in mind. I wanted Jenn to be involved with the families of her caretakers. I understood that I couldn't expect staff to keep her out and about every minute of the day; there would always be some down time when they would hang out at home. If at least some of that time were spent in the homes of her caregivers, she would experience more variety, stimulation, and socialization than if she remained in the group home.

Jenn didn't relate well to the other clients who lived at Squire. She seemed to consistently ignore them. I don't know why she behaved in this way. Perhaps they weren't interesting to her: They couldn't take her anywhere, do anything for her, or entertain her. Their disabilities limited them in being able to successfully interact with her. I could see she needed to be around a family with normal everyday interactions to feel a sense of belonging and purpose.

Questions, hurdles, and roadblocks all persisted as I worked to address these and other issues. Who was liable for workers' comp if staff were injured while caring for a client in their own home? What about state requirements regarding the number of nights a client could spend out of the group home before benefits were stopped? What were the rules regarding taking a client out of the country? I challenged all these questions and pushed against any limitations that would prevent me from giving Jenn the most normal and fulfilling life possible.

WHEN WE BROUGHT Jenn to Ability (Datahr), we brought someone with a unique communication disability and a new factor that wasn't previously available for their clients: a supplemental needs trust. The funding in this trust allowed for monetary benefits not available before its creation. Most families could not support the private staff, vehicle, and entertainment options without this new financial tool.

If you were a client with this particular kind of trust, you qualified for Medicaid. Other trusts didn't have this feature, and all your medical, housing, and treatment expenses would quickly drain those assets. Once the trust was depleted, the only spending money you had was the thirty-five-dollar-a-month Medicaid benefit after your primary care was covered. This small stipend had to be used for clothing, entertainment, and personal essentials. This left the burden of funding learning programs and community outings to the organization that, as a nonprofit, was stretched to their limit for funding essential client care through private donor dollars and money from tight state budgets. With the supplemental needs trust, Jenn was able to live a vastly more exciting and meaningful life than others in her disabled situation. We were moving into uncharted territory on the possibilities of how this trust could be used and paving the way for others who would come after us.

Chapter 6

A WAY TO PAY BACK

A few years after Jenn arrived at Ability (Datahr), I was asked to volunteer to do the "family segment" of recurrent training for their employees. I came in once every few months to speak to new personnel about my experiences as a client's family member.

Continued instruction for all employees was an ongoing theme in the organization, with workshops offered throughout the year. Ability recognized that family members could bring a different perspective to their staff and decided to include them in the mandated coursework they required for their employees.

The family segment of these classes gave employees the opportunity to ask questions of family members that normally would not be appropriate to ask. These included "Why don't some families come more often to visit their loved one?" Or "Why do families get so upset over trivial things like missing, discolored, or stained laundry?" These questions were brought up so often that I made discussion of them a regular part of my presentations.

It was important for employees to understand these answers so they wouldn't be wrongly judgmental toward the families they were serving. There were any number of answers to these questions, but after a lot of soul-searching, I offered some insights I thought would be helpful.

When I considered why someone's family might not come to visit as often as staff believed they should, one of my experiences offered what I thought served as an explanation. I had witnessed firsthand one such discrepancy with a family at Hillcrest.

There was a teenage girl at that rehab center who was in a vegetative state after a car accident and after many months showed no signs of improving beyond this point. She was an only child of a darling couple who, like us, came daily to see their daughter and oversee treatments in her recovery process.

As time passed and there was no change in their daughter, the parents began to have different ways of processing their pain and how they handled this tragedy. I watched as the mother came with comfy new clothing items for her daughter to wear and spent time doing her daughter's hair and nails. She talked to her daughter, read articles to her out of magazines and newspapers, and gave her words of encouragement. She would do this even though there was no response or visual clue that any of this was heard or processed, but this mother was not dissuaded. Her devotion was relentless, and I admired her for it.

By contrast, the father became so profoundly saddened and depressed by his daughter's condition that he found it more and more difficult to visit her. He talked to Mark and me various times about the feeling that in his mind she was dead; only the shell of her remained. "I just can't keep coming here and seeing her like this," he tearfully told us one day.

The father asked for a legal medical order to not resuscitate his daughter. The mother did not agree, asking instead that all possible medical intervention required be used to keep her daughter alive.

From that point on, the mother continued to visit her daughter each day, and on rare occasions the father came for a brief visit. His absence was not for lack of love. I understood it was because the pain of visiting was too overwhelming. For his own self-preservation and mental health, he had to refrain from frequent visits with his daughter.

I thought it was important for Ability employees to recognize that people handle pain in different ways and to be careful in making judgments of others who are suffering. I didn't want them to make assumptions without knowing the full story.

For the laundry question that employees often brought to my attention, I clearly understood this issue from my own experience with Jenn while she was living both at Hillcrest and Ability. White socks became pink, dark clothing came back splattered with bleach stains, and various articles sent to be washed never came back. For the parents and family members at both facilities, laundry issues became a focus—a pet peeve.

As one of those family members, I knew exactly why this simple thing was so upsetting. Our sons and daughters came to the organization with varying degrees of challenges and disabilities and we could do little to make them better. But laundry issues were a universal frustration for all the families, and something that seemed fixable to us.

To the staff, worrying about laundry seemed insignificant when considering all the things that go into a consumer's safety and care. They couldn't understand why families were so focused on something like pink socks and spent their energy complaining about this, when their loved one couldn't live independently because of their many disabilities.

I talked with them and explained that the atrophied limbs, behavior issues, low IQ, or loss of memory were of great concern to us, but those weren't things we could successfully have any effect on—laundry was.

Over the years, many employees told me that my session with them was the first time someone helped them to understand why people would be so upset about trivial things. Now they understood and could approach families in a more positive and reassuring way.

That employees could take a valuable lesson away from my sessions was a great reward for me, and I enjoyed giving something back to the organization that did so much for my family. The questions they asked gave me pause and stimulated my thinking through situations I had not considered before.

I heard from many staff within the Ability organization that the story of *pink socks* continues to be passed on to new hires. That kind of positive feedback was a huge compensation for the little time it took me to try to make a difference.

ABILITY BEYOND DISABILITY, was an organization that gave me the flexibility to create a meaningful life for my daughter. It was instrumental in enabling me to help Jennifer have a more normal life and build lasting relationships with her caregivers and their families. They gave me the opportunity to speak at the employee workshops, and because of that, I felt there was at least one positive outcome from Jenn's tragedy. Their staff was getting an insider's view by integrating some of my hard-earned lessons into their vast knowledge base to help them better serve their clients. I relished the thought and clung to it as a hopeful way to reconstruct my life after an accident brought me to a sudden and tragic place of despair.

Chapter 7

MARIA

Maria was among the earliest hires to be a personal one-on-one for Jenn. Aside from her full- time position as a caregiver, she was also a part-time student at the University of Connecticut, slowly working her way through college to be a social worker.

At twenty years old and standing a mere five foot two, Maria's short stature and youth did nothing to minimize her overall presence. With hazel eyes and medium brown hair, this sturdy girl would quickly prove to be confident, fearless, and have the endurance to work with a client who seemed to be in constant motion and into everything.

Training Maria was a work of joy, and building a relationship of trust and understanding came easily to us. Trust was key here. I would not only be entrusting my daughter's care into the hands of a young adult, but also providing a car for her to use and a credit card to pay for things. I knew it must have sounded like a cushy job, getting paid to do fun things with my daughter each day, but in reality it was far from that. Jenn was not always easy to work with, especially in those early days at the Ability organization.

She would be a challenge for any caretaker. With her frontal lobe brain injury, she lacked any sense of appropriateness. She was loud in public when happy or when being redirected. She was also compulsive and would do things like grab a handful of french fries from a stranger's plate as she passed by a patron in a restaurant, pick up a piece of already chewed gum off the floor, or rudely push people out of her way as she walked through stores or down a sidewalk. It was also not beyond her to approach a stranger and pick a piece of lint off their collar or even reach into their pocket to see if they had any treats like a piece of candy or gum. Jenn was inappropriate and unpredictable. To say that she was a handful was putting it mildly.

As if this weren't enough, she also made a repetitive droning noise when asked to do tasks or when being directed from one place to another, a shrieking moan that grated on the nerves. I don't know why she made this sound, but it did add yet another awkward element to being able to work with her, especially when Jenn got excited and her noise became loud and persistent.

Maria was dissuaded by none of this.

After spending two weeks working extensively with her on caring for Jenn, I knew she was ready to launch out on her own. I limited my visits to every other day, giving her freedom to explore some of the options she wanted to do with Jenn.

Maria told us she was determined to take Jenn to movies. Not understanding the dialog and therefore the plot, Jenn might laugh when others in the theater were weeping. Such was the case when they went to see *Titanic*. As bodies began floating in the iceberg-laden waters beside the sinking ship, Jenn started to laugh. "People started turning around and looking at us like, 'What's wrong with you, are you crazy?' Maria told me the next day with a giggle. "I just shrugged my shoulders, like I didn't know why she would do such a thing."

As I listened to Maria tell the story, I reflected on what my own emotional response would have been. I would have felt mortified, embarrassed, and disappointed that Jenn had made a scene. Mark and I were both sensitive to her inappropriate behaviors that we felt made us a spectacle in public. Try as we might, we couldn't find humor in behavior that called attention to her—and to us. I became acutely aware that for staff to view her actions as funny was a healthier way of reacting. For them to be the best companion for her, they needed to take situations like this lightly.

Over time, Maria learned which movies Jenn could follow and respond better to, but there would be many failed attempts before getting it right.

Maria loved to tell the story of the time Jenn threw her empty popcorn box at the person two rows in front of them.

"The person she hit turned around like, 'What just happened?' I mouthed the word 'Sorry' and shrugged my shoulders. What else could I do? What was really weird was it seemed that Jenn actually aimed at that person. It wasn't like she was just tossing her box away. Why she decided to do it is curious; maybe she just wanted to have some fun. We do this kind of joking around stuff at Squire, so maybe she was just mimicking that. Whatever her reason, I thought it was funny and the person in front didn't seem mad, just surprised."

Controlling all the unexpected behaviors that Jenn seemed to come up with daily, if not hourly, was not an easy task for a young person to take on, but Maria was up for the challenge and conducted herself way beyond her years as a professional and loving caregiver.

Maria would tell us of the times when Jenn did bring her to tears. More than once she discovered Jenn trashing her room. The bed was stripped, the closet emptied of makeup, clothes, learning materials (many having small pieces like puzzles), shoes, and jewelry in a jumbled heap. Every drawer was cleared, contents thrown into the pile. I saw Jenn's work on more than one occasion, so I knew it would take more than an hour to re-sort and put everything away.

After repeated "trashings," Mark engineered a lock for the double closet doors in Jenn's room so that future episodes would only involve the bed and drawers. This made her blitzes easier to clean up, and helped Maria feel more in control of her charge.

Then one day Jenn moved beyond whatever drove her to trash her room and replaced it with putting things away or getting them in order—another compulsive behavior.

She would put away anything left lying around. Jenn's idea of putting something away was stowing it out of sight: under the sofa cushions, in the garbage, under the bed, or under the seat of the car. She'd pour liquids down the sink unless she wanted to drink them, which meant that a container of coffee, orange juice, or milk would quickly be snatched up and dumped down the drain. Crumbs were brushed onto the floor, and tissues had to be pushed down in their box, not sticking up for the next user.

Jenn now liked items to be carefully lined up in horizontal or vertical rows. If you were working on an activity with her, all the crayons had to be in a straight line and the paper had to be perfectly aligned with the edge of the table. Shoes put under her bed at night were placed right next to each other with the toes pointing forward and no spaces in between.

Fixing other peoples' hair was another of Jenn's obsessions. All her staff, as well as Amy and I, had hair long enough to bother her if it hung down straight on the sides of our faces. To Jenn, that hair had to be put behind our ears. If a small piece moved from behind our ear, she was quick to stop us and put it back in its place. If she was across the room and spotted that loosely hanging hair, she would rush over to quickly replace it where she thought it belonged.

In some of these new behaviors I saw a glimmer of my former daughter who pre-accident was extremely neat and well organized. But it was still a little hard to accept that this was how those parts of her previous personality were presenting themselves.

It was physically challenging to care for Jenn. It was always a struggle steering her away from a restaurant if you were heading to a different destination, even if you'd just been there. Jenn's damaged brain didn't give her the normal "full" signal, so she was always ready to eat, even if she had just completed a meal.

Weakness was not one of Jenn's disabilities. Strong and mobile, she had to be watched all waking hours much like you would a two-year-old child. She didn't understand things like not walking out in front of cars, not touching a hot stove, or being careful not to slip on ice. She was also unaware of curbs, traffic lights, poisons, and other hazards in the world around her. When Jenn awoke from her coma, she was in a whole new world that had few references back to the one pre-accident. And like a two-year old, she was unable to express herself except with loud, harsh sounds and body language. This created frustration both in Jenn and those around her.

While she had relearned many things, some other skills didn't stick with her. Jenn learned to wash herself, with supervision, but because she didn't seem to understand the need to do it, would take a shortcut if she wasn't constantly supervised. A simple thing like brushing her teeth took years of continued training and she still didn't do a sufficient job to keep her teeth clean. This had to be done for her by personal staff while battling a strong and uncooperative client. Hyper-sensitive to touch, Jenn was a handful when it came to nail care, hair, teeth, bathing, drying, dressing, and applying lotions or cosmetics.

Jenn was forever creating what I perceived as uncomfortable situations requiring great courage for Maria to handle. At the same time, Maria was often tasked with reassuring people in the community, who didn't understand Jenn's idiosyncratic behavior, that all was okay. Because Jenn walked and was mobile, people didn't always recognize that she had a disability. When Maria anticipated crowded situations, she sometimes took Jenn out in a wheelchair to navigate her more easily around the throngs of people. The wheelchair was also a clear message to bystanders that Jenn was disabled and thus garnered fewer surprised looks from people.

Maria told us she loved the challenge of building a new life for Jenn and was focused on getting her out of the house and into the community. She became my pioneer when it came to experimenting with new kinds of events and activities. Because she could skillfully manage Jenn, she opened up a world of possibilities that enabled my daughter to live an adventuresome and exciting life, more than any of us had imagined.

During one of my visits to Squire, Maria presented me with a new idea.

"Is it okay for me to go up with Jenn in a private airplane at the local Danbury airport? I'm curious to see how well she would do with flying; maybe we can travel commercially someday."

My mind started spinning, thinking about how this would play out for Maria. I couldn't imagine how she could get Jenn into a little four-seater plane. There is a big step you must make while ducking under the wing to climb into the aircraft. How would Maria manage that? Would Jenn be disruptive during the flight, touching things she shouldn't or making too much noise? There seemed to be countless stumbling blocks that could make this a disaster and I didn't want that to happen. But I also didn't want to discourage new ideas, so I began strategizing with Maria about how this might work. She'd already checked out details with the general aviation flight service at the airport.

"They have a stool that would be used to help Jenn make the big step into the plane. The pilot who has agreed to take us will also be glad to help get Jenn up and into the back seat. They don't see that this would be an issue."

Another concern was whether the flight would make Jenn nauseated. "No worries," said Maria. "The pilot is prepared for that whenever he takes passengers up. They have baggies on board just like in the commercial airliners. But unlike a commercial flight, if Jenn were to get sick, we can just come back to the airport and land."

Maria was well prepared and had done her homework on how to create this adventure. I questioned whether it would work out but agreed for her to move forward with the plan.

Maria made the flight reservation, and the day after they flew, I got a full report.

"Jenn loved it!" Maria explained. "It took a little convincing for her to leave on the headset that is required in a private aircraft, but after a few initial attempts to remove it, she settled back and enjoyed the views. Looking out the window at the landscape sweeping out to the distant horizons below, brought on calm and positive head nods from Jenn. We could hear the airport tower and pilot talking in airplane-speak over our headsets which was really neat. They purposely put the mic of Jenn's headset toward the back of her head so if she made any noises, they wouldn't interfere with communications onboard.

"I sat in the front passenger seat but whenever I looked back at her, she was smiling and gave me a nod or one of her salutes."

Maria and I both knew Jenn would employ a little salute, like a single British royal hand wave, as her way of confirming she was okay, and all was well.

"We only had a one-hour flight, but during that time we were able to fly over Candlewood Lake, Danbury, and Brookfield. He also flew us over Squire Court so we could see it from the air. It was neat to see an aerial view of our familiar haunts."

The actual airtime was short, only thirty minutes, but the reward was huge. Now we knew Jenn could fly. In fact, she was a great passenger and as in other modes of transportation, it had a calming effect on her.

After this very successful experiment, Maria and Jenn flew commercially many times over the coming years and future caregivers continued the ritual.

IT WAS MARIA'S first summer working with Jenn, and she was looking for new ways to get them out to enjoy the warm weather. While having lunch together at our favorite sandwich shop, Maria offered her latest idea.

"If you are okay with it, I'd like to take Jenn out on a motorboat. They have rentals at nearby Candlewood Lake. I think she would enjoy doing this, especially because of the motion of the boat on the water."

I asked her, "Will you be able to manage her alone in a boat?"

"Sure, I can. Jenn is really good for me and cooperative when I show her new things," Maria reassured me.

"Okay, go for it," I agreed.

With my approval, plans were set in place for the following Wednesday and the weather was predicted to be perfect. Mark and I planned to visit that day, so we agreed to meet them dockside afterward.

The weather was ideal: blue skies, calm winds, and a temperature hovering around the eighty-degree mark.

Like other small lakes in the Northeast, Candlewood was surrounded by rolling forested hills that we could see on the opposite shoreline. This was a nice oasis from the hustle and bustle of Danbury proper and busy Interstate 84 that were hidden from view.

As we walked out on the dock to meet the boaters, the breeze carried the usual fishy smell that hinted at what was beneath the turbulent waters stirred up by the propellers of the approaching watercraft's motor. Right on schedule, their small boat inched its way toward us.

As the boat drew closer, we saw two happy, beaming girls on board as they prepared to dock. Mark helped Captain Maria secure the boat to the mooring while Jenn remained seated.

Jenn gave us one of her big, wide-open-mouth smiles and rapid waves—it was clear she was happy we had made the surprise appearance after her adventure. It was always fun to see her face when we appeared in unexpected places, doing a double take as if thinking, "Is that really my parents over there waiting for me?"

Once the boat was secured, Maria held Jenn's arm to help her up and out of the boat and couldn't wait to tell us about their experience and how much Jenn enjoyed herself. "I think Jenn's favorite part was taking off from the dock and coming back in because that was when the boat rocked the most—motion is always calming for her. She also seemed to really like going fast out in the middle of the lake with the wind blowing in her hair as she waved at other boaters we passed by."

Waving to people was something that Jenn did a lot. We didn't know if it was a gesture of acknowledgment, or if she was trying to be friendly. Whatever the reason, it was an endearing behavior and most often had a very positive effect on others, as they would respond by waving back and giving Jenn a big smile.

I couldn't think of a more perfect way for Maria and Jenn to spend a summer afternoon: out on the water, taking in the warm rays of the sun and feeling the breeze on their faces. I couldn't have been happier for my daughter. This was exactly the kind of enjoyable activity I wanted for her.

Local trips were fine, but Maria felt the need to adventure beyond the corridors of Danbury and Brookfield. She was determined to expose both herself and Jenn to new and exciting places farther away that required one or more overnight stays in a hotel. After much research on her part, she decided that they would travel to Block Island, just off the coast of Rhode Island, to try this idea out. Doing the typical touristy thing, she sent us a postcard from their vacation spot.

May 30, 1995
Greetings from Block Island!
The ferry ride was lots of fun— Jenn got a kick out of
all the rocking. The hotel was beautiful, but the weather
was very windy & wet. We went for a tour and explored
Mohegan Bluffs (where the Native Americans were pushed
over)—the bluffs are really high! Jenn had a great time and
so did I! Jennifer even went shopping. She went into several
stores without any prompting at all. Can't wait to get the
pictures back to show you. See you soon – Jenn & Maria

All went well on this trial run, so Maria began in earnest
to plan other road trips to a variety of destinations. But as
successful as these early adventures with Jenn were, it took
Maria becoming ill on one of their trips for us to realize it
was important to have two people travel with Jenn when they
were far from the group home.

When Maria came to work for Jenn, our daughter Amy
was in high school. Though she wanted to be involved with
her sister regularly, it was hard for Amy to find time to see
Jenn. To plan a trip for the two sisters to spend time together,
Maria decided they'd go to Washington, DC, during one of
Amy's school breaks so the threesome could take in all the
capitol had to offer. Things were set in place, and a few
weeks later we enjoyed receiving another postcard.

April 17, 1996
Hello, Hello! from Washington, DC.
Bill and Hillary Clinton were out of town for the weekend
so we all made our own fun. Jenn has kept us on our toes—
she's always reaching for a pocket or something! We visited
Lincoln, the White House, the Washington Monument,

*and a couple of museums at the Smithsonian, plus Old
Town Alexandria and Georgetown. Last night we went on
a cruise up the Potomac. It was very nice!! The train ride
was good—always someone or something to look at. See you
soon, Love Maria, Amy, and Jenn*

A year later, with the success of the Washington trip still
fresh in their memories, Maria planned a new and more
complex kind of travel for the three of them—a destination
that included both a plane ride and a cruise ship. Daring,
yes, but oh what a memorable time I knew they would have.

Maria made all the arrangements for their three-day
adventure. The first leg of their journey was a flight from
Newark to Miami where they boarded a Carnival cruise ship
heading to Nassau and Paradise Island in the Bahamas.

Amy and Maria told us that things generally went
well with the trip getting off to a good start as a friendly
Jamaican crew member cheered Jenn up the ramp from
the dock to the ship's main deck and got them comfortably
settled in their cabin. But as expected, there were also some
awkward moments along the way, especially in the dining
room. Jenn's inappropriate noise levels and lack of table
manners during meals caused fellow passengers to glare.
Although she no longer threw food, she would often try to
eat with her hands instead of utensils. Maria was quick to
redirect her and didn't seem to give it a second thought.
She pushed forward, determined to make their adventure
successful, and indeed it was. They reveled in the warm
climate and sandy beaches of the island paradise along with
the experience of having shared so many hours together on
the plane and ship. The stories of their trip were retold over
the years and reminded us of the true importance of two

sisters making a treasured memory after their childhoods were interrupted by tragedy.

WE RECEIVED MANY postcards over the years when Jenn went on her travels. Maria was adventuresome and enjoyed taking Jenn to new and interesting places as often as possible. She would put together itineraries that kept them busy and with camera in hand, documented every trip, showing Jenn in all sorts of places. Our daughter, who was very handicapped, seemed to be having a blast!

Maria's good nature, creativity, and dedication proved to be invaluable traits and would set the standard for all future hires. With her never-ending curiosity, she constantly thought outside the box and through careful trial and error was able to give Jenn a busy, active life.

These adventures were also Maria's way of introducing our family to the many possible things we could enjoy with our daughter: Disney World, swimming, boating, hiking, flying—there were no limits. She opened our eyes to the world of opportunities Jenn could explore. Maria's skillful, lighthearted redirections and carefree spirit helped strangers to not be alarmed by Jenn's odd behaviors. She did such a good job of orchestrating her excursions with Jenn, under the watchful eye of the public, that she helped them see how special a person with disabilities is and how to be tolerant of those who are different.

In far too short a time for me, Maria completed her college degree and was going to move on with her life. Before leaving, she trained other personal staff and set an example that would be used for all future caretakers who would carry on with her work. Maria continued to earn advanced degrees in her field of study, and later married, but she continued to be in contact with us over the years.

Unfortunately, Maria's life was cut short in a losing battle with cancer about ten years after leaving her position with Jenn. In her husband's eulogy, he talked about the work Maria favored most in her lifetime. It was deeply touching for us the hear that above all the community projects and organizations she had been involved with over the years, her favorite undertaking had been caring for Jenn.

Maria must have understood that she'd helped us find direction as we faced the daunting challenges of Jenn's TBI. She had taken a family shattered by tragedy and reset our compass toward a life filled with opportunities and encouragement. She changed our views of what Jenn could do and set the stage for a more positive and hopeful future. Maria accomplished this with a fearless determination, using all her creative talents and warm loving personality to demonstrate how someone with disabilities can and should have an exciting and rewarding life.

Chapter 8

CHRISTINE
AND SUZANNE

When we first walked into Squire with Jenn, we met Christine Boisvert, a member of the house staff. As we got to know her, we appreciated the special attention she gave to Jenn to help her adapt to the new environment.

Despite the fact that the staff were new at working with Jenn, within the first couple of weeks, Jenn and others in the group home went for an overnight trip to Washington, DC. Ability residents traveled in company vans to join a nationwide march in support of Americans with disabilities.

Chris later confided, "What were we thinking, taking this new client who was nonverbal on an overnight trip to a distant city when we didn't know or understand her?"

Once Chris pointed this out to me, I looked back at what my mindset was that I allowed my daughter to go on that trip. I desperately wanted Jenn to be able to go places and do things that had not been possible for more than a year. I wanted to believe that the camaraderie that would be a part of the adventure would benefit her. I did a lot of wishful thinking back then, always weighing the positive outcomes of her participation against the risks of potential harm. I forced myself to not be paralyzed with fear because I recognized that having her do nothing was just as harmful.

As trip preparations were made, I was reassured when I heard the ratio of clients to staff.

"We have as many staff going as residents," Chris told me. "There will be plenty of eyes to keep track of Jenn. We have to be even more watchful of her because she is more mobile than our wheelchair clients."

As I'd hoped, the excursion went smoothly, and Jenn successfully went on her first big trip since the accident. How much benefit she derived from the experience was not something that could be measured. But for me, it seemed positive for Jenn to take a first step forward without my full oversight. I don't know if it was more liberating for her or for me—I'd like to think that we shared that feeling equally.

WHEN WE HIRED Maria as personal staff, she and Chris quickly became best friends and often pooled their efforts to take the Ability clients who lived at the Squire group home out for fun adventures. Maria saw few barriers in taking everyone at Squire to functions like track meets, basketball games, state fairs, or even the Medieval Times dinner theater in Lyndhurst, New Jersey. She thought it was beneficial for the whole house to go to interesting places whenever possible instead of just Jenn and her on their own. Many of these trips were free, and others were paid for by the Ability organization. Chris agreed with Maria's ideas to get everyone away from their usual routines to do something different and exciting.

Maria loved telling me about the successful times they shared on those outings. One of her most proud accomplishments was when they went to the Massachusetts Big E State Fair for the first time.

"Right after breakfast we loaded all the staff and clients either in Jenn's car or the Ability van. Between the two vehicles, we got all the wheelchairs and everyone in. Once all clients were secured and on board, we headed to Springfield, Massachusetts, an hour-and-a-half drive from Squire. Everyone had a great time on the rides, eating corn dogs and cotton candy, and checking out the other attractions. There weren't any real problems during the day—there was plenty of staff to push the wheelchairs through the crowds or assist the walking clients, helping them navigate through the maze of the big fairway.

"Jenn had such a good time. She had one meltdown when her cotton candy was gone, and we were still eating ours. She began crying and whining as she watched us. I just had to get her somewhere else until they finished. She calmed down right away when I walked her over to an arcade, and we threw some basketballs at small hoops, though prizes were impossible to win. But that didn't matter; mission accomplished, Jenn was back to her happy-go-lucky self."

The Big E, also known as the Eastern States Exposition, proved to be so successful it became an annual outing for Squire. Billed as "New England's greatest state fair," it is the largest agricultural event on the East Coast and the seventh largest fair in the nation. I was pleased to hear how successful it was for Jenn and everyone involved.

WITHIN A SHORT time of Jenn's arrival at Squire, Chris moved into the assistant manager position at the group home, but that was soon to change. Later we reminisced about how things evolved. "When Maria and I started doing trips with the whole house," she explained, "I began to see how amazing it could be to work with Jenn and make a difference in one person's life. I did a lot of soul-searching when a one-on-one staff opening came up for Jenn and decided to leave my management position to become one of her personal caregivers, a decision I never regretted."

Serendipitously, Suzanne Benz was hired to fill Christine's position as assistant house manager. With a college degree in social work, Suzanne was a good placement in the management role.

"But like Christine," Suzanne shared with me, "I soon saw the advantages that came with being Jenn's one-on-one. You could have a huge impact on someone's life doing this job. In my management position, there was a lot of paperwork, not as much hands-on interaction with the clients, and I was confined to the group home. Chris and Jenn could get out and do interesting things. There was also the attractiveness of the scheduling and flexibility of hours that came with Jenn's position, and I loved that idea."

I was concerned that Ability would not be happy with Suzanne's decision to relinquish her management position to become another private staff for Jenn, and Suzanne confirmed my suspicions. "They told me they didn't understand why I would make a move to a lower paying position, especially when Jenn was so hard to work with. They tried to convince me not to make the change, but my mind was made up."

LUCKY FOR US, Chris and Suzanne, like Maria, were creative, hardworking, dedicated, and full of energy. They not only became the primary staff for Jenn, they also built an endearing three-way friendship as coworkers and client.

Chris, the fair blonde, and Suzanne, with her dark hair and olive skin, were like bookends for Jenn, who fell in the middle, with light brown hair and skin tones leaning toward Suzanne's. Like so many things that changed for Jenn after the accident, her naturally blonde hair had darkened to a soft brunette. All three girls were in their early twenties, full of youthful enthusiasm and zest for life.

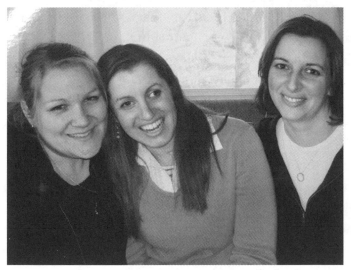

Chris, Jenn, and Suzanne.

JENN HAD MANY wonderful caregivers over the years, and we're forever indebted to them and appreciative of all they did for our family, but there was something different about Chris and Suzanne that set them apart from the rest. These two girls made the extraordinary move of bringing

Jenn into their homes and including her in their private lives. Jenn was at their homes so often that she became an integral part of their families.

The other important factor was that Chris and Suzanne became best friends, so they brought their two families together outside of work, adding their kids and spouses into the mix. This was the main ingredient in what would become a lasting bond between these two families and ours. In Chris and Suzanne's minds, the plan was for the three girls to be best friends forever. "We'll be three old ladies who, decades from now, will be going out for lunch in our purple dresses and red hats," they would tell me.

Mark and I weren't old, but when you have a child with special needs, you worry about aging and facing your mortality when your loved one is so dependent upon you. Amy reassured us that she would always be there for her sister. We were glad for that, but I understood that she would not always be as free as I was to oversee Jenn's care. Who knew where Amy would be living in the future? And if Amy was lucky enough to have a family, they would need most of her time. With Chris and Suzanne in Jenn's life, Mark and I began to see a possible future for Jenn when our time on this earth was over.

The level of trust we were developing with these girls was liberating. There was a deep sense of peace and calm within us where for the past few years we'd had only chaos. Listening to Chris and Suzanne talk about how they saw their future with Jenn was proof that the time and energy I'd spent advising and training them had paid off. This was the reward for my years of effort and was far beyond anything I could have ever hoped for. But I still had my work cut out for me in regard to Jenn. I wasn't hanging up my hat yet.

MOST DAYS IT was just Chris or Suzanne alone with Jenn, but there were special adventures that required at least two staff to accompany her. Christmas shopping was such a time. The three of them would slip away from their families and travel five hours by car to an outlet shopping mecca in Maine to collect gifts for the holiday. The overnight excursion wasn't just about the purchase of gifts; it was more about sharing time together, joking around, being silly, eating, venting about daily stresses, taking in local attractions, and mostly just having a fun outing.

Boxes and bags of every sort came back with them to Connecticut, along with photos recording little bits and pieces of how the girls made a wonderful memory out of something so simple as a shopping spree. Chris and Suzanne shared stories of the expected and unexpected in colorful detail. "We were at the counter of the CVS buying some shampoo when Jenn grabbed a Snickers candy bar, ripped the wrapper off, and snarfed down half of it in one gulp. We paid for it, Barb, no worries."

"Our first night there, we got a call from the hotel receptionist telling us they had a complaint from the people next door about our noise level," Chris said, laughing.

Suzanne quickly piped in, "And Jenn wasn't the culprit— it was Chris who was being loud, not her." All this was said in a joking way. The two girls loved to tease each other. It was all part of the banter that kept them, Jenn, and me endlessly entertained.

"It was only eight o'clock, not like anyone was sleeping. I saw those people next door— grumpy old farts," was Chris's defense.

"Because we got in early, we decided to let Jenn take a mega bubble bath in the room Jacuzzi. Jenn must have thought she was in heaven," Suzanne said.

Chris chimed in, "We put on her bathing suit so we could take pictures and then let her soak for about thirty minutes before dragging her out. Oh, my God, she didn't want to leave the warm water; we literally had to pull her out."

Looking at the photos of Jenn's Jacuzzi experience, I saw true pleasure written all over her face. She had a smile from ear to ear and was giving a big wave as though to say, "Look at this amazing and wonderful place these girls brought me to."

The bubbles were about a foot above the water surface as they cascaded over the sides of the tub and dripped from Jenn's body. The girls added a puff of foaming bubbles on her head to add humor to the scene.

But for Chris and Suzanne, the best story they brought home from the shopping adventure came from the night they were at a restaurant and the only seating available to them was at the bar.

Suzanne began the saga. "So, there was this guy at the bar sitting next to Jenn and he starts to talk with her. He was so trying to pick her up. As he talked, Jenn nodded her head and was smiling, even gave one of her sputtering laughs which just encouraged him. He kept talking and talking as Chris and I just sat watching, trying not to laugh out loud, even though it was hilarious. After a few minutes, he leans around Jenn and tells us that he thinks our friend has had too many drinks."

"Yep, you're probably right," Chris chimed in.

Their voices grew louder and more excitable with each segment of the story, and their animated gestures, batting eyelashes, and rolled eyes simulated the scene at the bar.

"Barb, it was hysterical to sit and watch this interaction. Jenn almost seemed flirtatious. He was a hot looking guy who'd had a few too many himself," Suzanne continued. "After a while, he got up and left. Maybe he thought Jenn wasn't going for his pickup line, so he moved on."

"Or he left before he passed out," Chris threw in.

This tale was retold countless times over the years with the flavor of casting Jenn as a magnet for roving young male eyes when the girls were out in public.

Chris and Suzanne loved watching young men take notice of Jenn. They always made sure she looked her best with nice clothes, well-styled hair, makeup, and jewelry—a pre-accident requisite for any outfit. Jenn was beautiful, resembling Jessica Alba, the actress, with her infectious smile and the same giddy twinkle in her eyes. It wasn't until guys took a closer look at her that they began to see that something wasn't quite right.

Over time, the girls collected countless stories from their outings. The best tales were retold for weeks, months, and years to come, testimony to how uniquely Chris and Suzanne viewed the world with Jenn as their charge. I can think of nothing that would have made Jenn feel more like a normal person than being off on a lark as a part of this threesome.

BOTH CHRIS AND Suzanne came to the job with husbands and young families: Chris had twin baby boys, Ian and Aaron. Suzanne had two daughters: Mary, in elementary school, and six-month-old Dianna. Both women would slowly weave "Aunt Jenn" comfortably into their family lives in a profound and loving way, and our daughter was a huge benefactor of the whole arrangement.

As the years passed by, new little ones arrived. Suzanne had Jackson, and Chris followed with Lily. Jenn was among the first visitors to see the girls in the hospital after each delivery. She also made many home visits during their time off to check on the new babies and their moms. When I took her to visit them, it was easy to see how excited she was to be with her beloved friends. Sitting as close as possible to them on the sofa, her face inches away from theirs, she laughed, giggled, and lovingly adjusted their hair. The new infant was of little interest to Jenn as she positioned herself so she could be right in the new mother's face, sucking up every bit of attention she could get. I understood that this was Jenn's way of showing her affection for them—she must have missed them terribly and anxiously awaited their return.

FOR ALL OF Chris and Suzanne's children, Jenn was in their lives as far back as their memories went. One day, I asked Suzanne's daughter, Mary, who had just turned nine, if she remembered a time when Aunt Jenn wasn't around. She was quick to reply, "Aunt Jenn's always been there. I know she lives in a group home, but she spends a lot of her time at my house."

"What does Aunt Jenn do at your house?" I asked.

"She and Mom cook dinner and do the dishes. She helps fold laundry, and we make a lot of cupcakes together. Even when we're in school, Mom and Aunt Jenn are busy doing things together."

"What kinds of things, Mary?"

"Oh, they do stuff like take Aunt Jenn's laundry to the cleaners or go grocery shopping. Umm, they also pick me up from school and sometimes drop me off at a friend's house, or we just go back home."

Christine's kids had similar stories about the daily routines their mom shared with Jenn.

I talked to seven-year-old Ian and Aaron one day when they came to Squire. "Ian, what do you think mom and Aunt Jenn do all day while you're in school?"

"I don't know, maybe clean Aunt Jenn's room and go shopping."

"What do you think, Aaron?" I asked.

"I think they work on papers, go out to eat with you, and maybe go to the car wash. Oh, yeah, Mom has to give Aunt Jenn a shower in the morning too. She's really loud when Mom does that."

"What does Aunt Jenn do at your house when she's there?"

"She and Mom cook dinner, and we play games with her while Mom cleans up." Ian offered.

I realized their saying Jenn helped Mom in preparing dinner was a stretch. As young children, they didn't see that Jenn's help consisted of hovering over Chris's shoulder and stirring a pot or pouring ingredients into a bowl. To them, it must have seemed that if two adults were in the kitchen as dinner preparations were underway, both adults shared equally in the tasks.

"Mom likes for us to show her our stuff," Aaron added.

"What kind of stuff?"

"Oh, things like our Legos and action characters. Mom sits her on the floor so she can reach everything, and we let her play with whatever she wants. She likes to use our markers too; she just scribbles but that's okay. And she likes to throw things—like a ball or wad of paper. You know the wrapper on a straw? Mom showed her how to blow the end off at someone and she likes to do that with us too."

"Yeah, Mom bought a whole box of straws just for us to play with Aunt Jenn," Ian added.

This was a normal family life Jenn could not attain on her own but enjoyed as a result of becoming part of the Benz and Boisvert families. It was as typical a life as anyone could ask for a young woman, aside from a nine-to-five work schedule. Although Ability had work options for their clients, that didn't seem an appropriate placement for Jenn. The mundane tasks that were rewarding and challenging for many other clients would not have held Jenn's attention or interest. It was far more stimulating for her to be actively involved with the Benz and Boisvert families.

THERE'S NOTHING LIKE a snow day in Connecticut. When the forecast calls for a winter storm, all children look forward to the day off from school, and Jenn's extended families were no different. With great anticipation, everyone in the household speculated about how many inches of the white stuff would fall. Would they get the whole day off or only have a late start? Those unscheduled reprieves from homework, tests, and getting up early to catch the school bus make snow days all the more special for kids, but a headache for most working parents as they scramble to find babysitters.

"It is so amazing to not have to worry about snowstorms now that I work with Jenn," Suzanne said. Chris said the same thing many times over the years. When the forecast was bad, one of them would call to tell me who was taking Jenn to their house for an overnight, so they'd be home for their kids the next morning. Later I'd hear the stories about how everything worked out.

"When it's storming outside, it's family time and Jenn joins right in with the cooking, cleaning, and watching cartoons or movies," Suzanne said. "She even occasionally gets

in the middle of the scrapping between her 'adopted' nieces
and nephews."

"Mom, Aunt Jenn cheated!" was a common refrain. The
children were too little to understand why this adult didn't
abide by the rules as they played things like Connect Four.
We'd worked with Jenn on how to play this game: taking
turns and trying to get four in a row before her opponent.
But turn-taking was a hard concept for her to understand.
She seemed to think the task was simply to get all the discs
in the holder. We consistently had to push her hand away
until after we dropped our disc in the frame, or she would
put all hers in and put the game away. And of course, that
was exactly what she did when playing with either Chris or
Suzanne's kids.

Lily often called out, "Mom, Aunt Jenn isn't taking turns!"

"You have to show her how to take turns, she doesn't
know how," Chris would try to console her youngest. But
sometimes, no amount of consoling would appease a frustrated three-year old.

"Yes, she does! She just wants to win," Lily would scream
as she stomped off to her room.

For Jenn, the more the kids whined or cried, the funnier
she seemed to think it all was. The bigger Lily's reaction,
the more Jenn laughed, and the madder Lily got. Jenn
didn't intend to upset the little ones—the fussing was just
extremely entertaining to her.

"But Lily loves Aunt Jenn," Chris explained to me, "so
after she has a hissy fit and storms off, she always comes back
and is then willing to help her learn how to play the game
the right way."

All this would take place in the house as the snowstorm
raged outside. Once the weather cleared, it was time for

sledding, making snow angels, and snowball fights. Everyone went outside and played in the new-fallen fluff, which entertained the troops. Jenn would be outside with them, even though she wasn't a big fan of the cold and wet. She seemed keen to watch all the commotion and would gladly throw a snowball someone handed to her but didn't want to get hit with one.

If Jenn were at Suzanne's house during a snowstorm, Jackson liked having someone sit on the floor with him and play with his Lincoln Logs, Legos, or other wooden construction toys. Once Jenn was helped to get down on the floor, she was more than willing to play with him. With careful dexterity, she would either line the blocks up in a perfect row or begin to build her own tower just as Jackson was adding pieces to his.

There wasn't any cheating when it came to this activity, so this little boy and Aunt Jenn could play without issue until sister Dianna came along to stir up mischief. Suzanne would shake her head when she told me what would happen.

"Of course, Dianna had to knock Jackson's tower down. So, while Jackson was crying, banging his fists and screaming at Dianna, and she was screaming back at him, Jenn was cracking up."

"She loves when my kids go after each other. When I see how she reacts to the fits, screaming, and crying, it helps me to keep my sanity. If that makes Jenn happy, maybe it isn't so bad. I love when she's laughing so hard that tears run down her cheeks, her nose starts running—which of course she wipes all over her shirtsleeve—and she can hardly catch her breath. How can I not be okay when I see poor Jenn sitting in the middle of it all, doubled over from laughing so hard. It helps me get through the day."

SLOWLY AND STEADILY, Jenn was weaving her way into the hearts of the Benz and Boisvert families. What started out as an unprecedented experiment for the Ability facility, a caregiver taking a client home, was proving to be the perfect way for my daughter to have an interesting daily routine for herself. But more importantly, she was also developing a support group of loving people she was comfortable with, and whom I could trust with her life.

Chapter 9

BONDING

As with all families, there are special occasions to mark milestones in life. These occasions were an important part of the Boisvert and Benz families, and Aunt Jenn was always on the guest list. Jenn's own family living in our area consisted of just Amy, Mark, and me, so we were happy she had a huge extended family through Chris and Suzanne. When the Boisverts or Benzes celebrated any special event, Aunt Jenn was there—graduations, dance recitals, basketball practice, sweet sixteen parties, Fourth of July festivities, and even major holidays. Everyone expected her to come.

Although I loved encouraging her involvement with all these dear people, it became important for me to also work on connecting Jenn's real family to her newly adopted ones.

We started this bonding process by having a big birthday party at the group home for Jenn each year and inviting Chris, Suzanne, and their families to join us. Amy came from wherever she was in her life— high school, college, or from New Jersey with her own family in later years. Many past caretakers continued to be a part of Jenn's world and were also invited. In total, there were about thirty attendees, which included the other residents and staff.

Often there was snow during her February birthday party. The spacious backyard had a decent slope, and when it was covered with snow, everyone wanted to take advantage of the welcome winter activity it offered. Plastic trash bags and sheets of cardboard from pizza boxes made perfect sleds for racing down the hill. Even Jenn seemed thrilled by the swift glide down the slippery slope with someone sharing the ride with her, but she was not a big fan of the trudge back up to the top.

A dinner of ham with all the fixings was prepared at Squire for the feast that evening. Jenn and all the kids hovered around the decorated cake sitting on the counter until their dinner plates were filled. After our tasty meal, it was time for cake. We sat Jenn at the kitchen table, and everyone gathered to sing "Happy Birthday" as she blew out the candles.

Balloons, streamers, laughs, food, and friends all made the party memorable each year as we celebrated Jenn's birthday. Having everyone gathered with us made the day special and was a vital first step in getting our families to bond.

THE BIRTHDAY PARTIES helped to connect our families, but that celebration was only once a year, and we needed more times to connect. What better way to bring us all together than to rent a beach house by the ocean for a week? I chose Ocean City, New Jersey, as the most family-oriented place for our group. Once I had everyone's approval, I started making plans for this adventure.

Chris and Suzanne would bring all their kids, but unfortunately the dads would be unable to come due to their work schedules. The girls would be paid as though it were a regular work week, like a working vacation. I rented a house close to the beach, and all was set in place when the time for our July reservation finally rolled around.

As our vacationers arrived at our beach destination, the ruckus of unpacking and claiming beds and rooms had Jenn in a spin trying to decide where to go next. Her loud voice of excitement added to the din that seemed to bounce off the walls and echo throughout the two-story residence.

The house teemed with kids and adults all under one roof during the fun-filled stay at the Jersey shore. Days were spent at the beach digging in the sand, lounging on chairs and blankets, talking, and joking around. The older kids and adults surfed the waves.

Locked in a vice grip with someone on either side of her, we walked Jenn to the water's edge and let the cool ocean waves splash on her legs. She squealed in delight as each wave seemed to surprise and enchant her.

Sandwiches, snacks, drinks, and fruit were prepared before leaving the beach house to keep hunger at bay until the late afternoon when we would be returning home. The sea gulls at the Jersey shore are aggressive about stealing food, and it wasn't unusual to have a sandwich or chip bag snatched right out of our hands.

Jenn didn't know to protect herself from the flying dive-bombers. At first, we tried just shooing the birds away from her, but there were so many, and they were so persistent, this defense didn't work. We finally got smart and resorted to using one of our large beach towels as a makeshift shelter to hide her from the overhead invaders.

It worked! With all the commotion and barricades we created, the birds kept away, and Jenn was never a victim of their tactics.

After returning from the beach and taking showers, everyone pitched in to prepare our evening meal. Someone would be in charge of the hamburgers and hot dogs on the grill while others made the side dishes of typical summer fare: potato salad, baked beans, corn on the cob, and garden salad. After eating, we worked together to quickly clean up, so we could go off for our evening activities.

We headed to the mini golf course, ice cream parlor, or amusement park in nearby Wildwood. With all age levels in tow, Mark and I volunteered to watch the toddlers as the older kids and adults, including Jenn, wanted to give all the rides a go.

In a couple of hours, everyone was exhausted and ready to head home for bed. We were quite the weary bunch as we dragged ourselves back to the beach house, but the next day, everyone was up early and excited to do it all over again.

One morning we rode bikes on the boardwalk. There were single bikes for adults and older kids, and a carriage bike for one of us to take the small kids and Jenn in. Try as we might, we could not get Jenn to do her share of pedaling in the carriage bike. She took in all the sights just like the little ones, without doing any of the work. Quite a caravan of pedalers we were as we headed down the boardwalk for about an hour. Jenn loved it.

A fond memory of our early Ocean City retreats still brings a chuckle when we think about it. Everyone was ready to start walking to the beach. Chris and Suzanne had Jenn in her swimsuit, sunscreen applied, leg brace and shoes on, all set to go. The kids were very little and required an adult to apply their sunscreen—that was my job. We had loaded up the paraphernalia for a day at the beach: towels, beach chairs, shovels, coolers, toys, and umbrellas.

Everyone started heading to the door but Jenn. "She won't walk!" Chris said with a puzzled look on her face.

"Come on Jenn, let's go," Suzanne encouraged as both she and Chris tried to nudge her along, but Jenn wasn't moving.

"Okay, something's wrong. Maybe her sock or insole is bunched up, or the brace isn't on right—something must be bothering her," Chris said. She and Suzanne removed her shoes to see what was wrong. Well, it wasn't the sock, the brace, or the insole.

"I can't believe it, look at this," Suzanne exclaimed as she held up a plastic canister of camera film. "This was in the toe of her shoe."

"What! How did that get there?" Chris questioned. "Jenn this is your greatest 'Kodak moment' ever."

By now all of us were laughing so hard we could hardly breathe. Although I doubt Jenn understood what was so funny, she joined in with our laughter adding her loud and high-pitched happy voice to the hysteria that encompassed the room. We figured that in the commotion of preparing everyone for the beach, Jenn had ended up with an unusual addition to her footwear.

Ocean City was an annual event fully paid for by the trust. It was one of the many beneficial things those funds offered her, bringing caregivers and families together to strengthen bonds of friendship. Best of all, she had the time of her life during those magical weeks in Ocean City. Although she wasn't a big fan of walking in the sand or having sunscreen applied, she actively engaged with all those around her with hugs, laughs, friendly nudges, games, rides, and shared days in the sun.

Of equal importance, everyone in Jenn's three families got to know and care for each other. We each had our moments of frustration or fatigue. We saw each other drag into the kitchen each morning in our pajamas, without makeup or combed hair. For a week, we were living together and working as one large family. I was happy to experience the extended family life Jenn enjoyed with Chris and Suzanne. My heart glowed as I saw how warmly and lovingly everyone interacted with Jenn. She wasn't set aside or ignored but instead was an integral part of everything going on with the kids and adults. I saw that life was good for her around these people.

These gatherings were exhausting and exhilarating, but there is no better way to connect with people than to actually do something with them. Working and playing together at the beach house bonded all of us. That was exactly what I wanted.

IT'S HARD TO have humor in a family where tragedy has struck. Even as the years rolled past, we couldn't escape the reality that Jenn's disabilities had altered her life's path and ours. It was difficult at times to see the bright side of life, and we needed the coping tool of laughter to save our family from total despair.

It was such a blessing that Chris and Suzanne accepted Jenn as she was when she arrived at Squire. They were not burdened with trying to constantly fix her and return her to her former self. Instead, they came to work prepared to have as much fun as they could and keep Jenn happy and enjoying the day. These two young women both had a great sense of humor. They played off each other like a dual comedy team that kept all of us entertained. Sometimes it seemed like a vaudeville routine when they were together. They innocently and unknowingly brought a lighter side of things back into our often dark and humorless lives.

Post-accident Jenn loved slapstick. For her, few things were funnier than watching someone trip, flailing their arms and legs in all directions to prevent falling. This awkward action on the part of some unsuspecting victim would put Jenn in stitches. Aware of this, staff would pretend to trip as they walked along just to get a reaction from her. Chris and Suzanne were masters at this pretended tripping motion and would use that trick whenever Jenn was in a bad mood.

Playing a practical joke on Joe, the group home manager, was always fodder for a good laugh. I knew Joe to be an agreeable, good-natured person. Born in Portugal and brought to this country as a young child, his dark hair and warm skin tones hinted at his Lusitanian heritage. He had a solid and sturdy build and was strong as an ox. His round face sported a small beard which outlined his jawline, giving him a clean-cut look. Thank goodness for his even temperament, as his limits would be endlessly tested by his two coworkers.

"Hey Joe, Mark and Barbara are concerned that Jenn might accidentally get locked in the trunk of her car. There is a safety pull-tab, but we don't know if it really works or if Jenn would be able to use it to get out if we train her how to do it. Will you help us try this out?" Chris and Suzanne explained to him.

"Sure, if it worries Mark and Barb, we have to reassure them. Let's give it a try," Joe willingly offered.

Exactly how Jenn was accidentally going to get herself locked in the trunk didn't seem to cross Joe's mind. His only thought was that if the Rubins had this safety concern, it needed to be tested. So, into the trunk went Joe. Once the girls closed the lid, locking him inside, he found that locating the emergency pull-tab in the dark wasn't as easy as he expected.

"Chris, I can't find the tab, I can't see." He was met with silence.

"Suzanne, do you guys hear me? I can't get out.

"Are you guys there? Open the trunk!" he began to plea.

I could imagine how it was for him as he called out to the girls to open the trunk, and the only sound he heard was the beating of his own heart as his voice echoed in the dark. Finally, Joe began to question what they had asked of him. Was this another one of their pranks? His questioning was confirmed by the absolute uproar as the girls couldn't hold back their laughter any longer. One thing for sure, Joe knew the girls had gotten him once again with one of their practical jokes.

Another time, Joe went into his office and found that everything was wrapped in newspaper: the stapler, all the pens, the calculator, the chair, everything on the desk. Knowing Joe would be in meetings for a good part of the day, the girls had plenty of time to complete their project. Jenn loved using Scotch tape and happily played her part by enthusiastically securing each item in its newspaper wrapping. True to his good nature, he took it in stride with a chuckle as he walked into his office and began opening each of the carefully secured packages.

More than once, when he went out to his car in the driveway, he would find it wrapped in toilet paper, the rolls thrown over the top and underneath by Jenn and her accomplices to encapsulate the entire vehicle. Joe was a good sport about it and told me, "I look at these pranks as a team-building exercise and a great way to de-stress from everyday routines."

AFTER JENN'S ACCIDENT, we became very aware of safety ratings and the importance of curb weight of the cars for our family. "Abe Lincoln" would serve as a funny catch phrase for Chris and Suzanne when it came to the vehicle we chose for Jenn's purposes. The Lincoln brand was a little over-the-top for our young drivers, but we needed to keep them safe and wanted the heaviest, most crashworthy car available. At that time, the Lincoln Town Car was the clear choice.

A used Lincoln was in our price range, but the luxury brand gave Suzanne and Chris pause—it wasn't what a twenty-year-old would choose and seemed like a cumbersome mode of transportation. So, to make light of an otherwise awkward situation, the car became fondly known as Abe Lincoln. Our first Abe Lincoln was a 1992, silver-gray, 4200-pound behemoth with the boxy design of the time.

"This car is so long! Its hood is so far out there I don't even know where it ends," Chris told me. "My car is half this size."

I could see her point. It was a tank of a vehicle, the only thing bigger on the road was an eighteen-wheeler!

We had several Abe Lincolns over the years, and the safety features kept improving with newer models. No matter how many times we traded in Jenn's car, she always recognized her Abe Lincoln and would dart right for it in a parking lot, even though the color may have changed. Sometimes she would sit inside Abe when it was parked in the driveway of the group home. We were never sure if this was a hint that she was ready to go or if she just needed some down time away from all the hustle and bustle going on inside the house.

After twelve years of Lincolns, the girls finally had enough of driving around in what to them looked like a limo and convinced us to consider another brand for our next replacement vehicle.

"Barb, Honda's SUV would be great for winter conditions and the safety ratings and weight are the same as the Lincoln. I think all of us would rather drive one of those instead of Abe," Suzanne explained.

She was right. Once we checked out all the details of this new option, it seemed like a good idea, and we made the change. The girls were happy, but unfortunately Jenn never recognized her car after that point. The gray Honda must have looked just like all the other cars in the parking lot, and because of that, she would head to the first available vehicle that she came to and try to get in. That required staff to constantly redirect her until they reached the Honda.

"I think she truly misses Abe!" Chris sadly announced one day.

JOKING AROUND, GIVING big belly laughs, and having a good time was just a part of Chris and Suzanne's nature. Their infectious humor carried over when bringing Jenn out in public. I think their candid way of looking at the odd behaviors Jenn exhibited in the community helped strangers feel comfortable around Jenn and generally tolerant of her inappropriate ways.

I remember the many times I was with Chris or Suzanne when they brought Jenn into a public restroom. How would I react if I were a stranger who came into a restroom where a young woman was making loud noises in the handicapped stall? It would be alarming, and I would probably leave. But with the gentle banter from the other woman in the stall, it was obvious that one of them had special needs.

"Hurry up Jenn, I have to go too."

"Hold my hands, I don't want you touching anything in here."

"Don't open the door Jenn, and face toward me."

"Don't walk out yet, you have to wait!"

"Jenn you have to move over that way for me to open the door. More, more, I can't get the door open."

Their voices could be heard behind the handicapped door as Jenn laughed through the whole process.

I never witnessed anyone fleeing the restroom, and I saw countless women come into the area with children in tow, explaining, "Everything is okay, it's just a special person." I appreciated the kind way they referred to someone who was challenged with physical or mental issues. "A special person" was exactly the term Chris and Suzanne used to describe Jenn. I loved that choice of terminology instead of other labeling words that had a more negative tone.

There were many occasions when people in public places could have become alarmed by our daughter's peculiar behaviors, like when she had a fit because they didn't enter a restaurant or when she was uncontrollably laughing about some mundane thing that others didn't notice. But Chris and Suzanne's jovial, lighthearted way of moving her on or coaxing her to calm down were a clear signal to others that nothing was amiss.

WHEN JENN WAS timid or anxious about a situation, she fed off Chris and Suzanne's laughter and seemed to understand their body language as an indication that all was okay. She needed this reassuring support when Chris and Suzanne wanted to take her on a roller-coaster ride.

They knew Jenn had enjoyed roller coasters pre-accident and liked other rides at the Big E State Fair. Even so, it required some pretty creative antics to get her into the tight safety seats of this attraction. Mark and I watched from the sidelines at Wildwood as the girls approached the platform. Jenn was excited and happy at first, but stepping from the platform into the seat presented a problem. Suzanne got in the car first and carefully guided Jenn over the uneven surface while Chris maneuvered her from the back.

"Come on Jenn, we've got ya," they encouraged. Lots of giggles and horsing around were the grease that finally got Jenn to seamlessly glide into the car. Once seated, it was obvious that she was not happy with the restraints that secured her—too much touching, and she was not thrilled to have her right arm lifted and belts adjusted around her torso. Her voice rose above the noisy carnival din as she let it be known that she was more than a bit disgusted with the initial protocol that was required.

Secured in her seat, once the motion of the roller-coaster began, Jenn relaxed and joined in the screams and laughter throughout the high-speed ride. As they came whipping around the tight curve near where I was standing, pure pleasure was spread across Jenn's face. She was laughing with her head tilting on Suzanne's shoulder as the momentum of the ride pushed her closer to her friend. Her loud squeals matched those of her friends and other riders. After that introduction, gentle roller coasters became a favorite of Jenn's at any state fair or carnival. She would always eagerly approach these rides and join in the fun with her compadres.

The humor exhibited by Chris, Suzanne, and previously Maria, was healing for our family as I'm sure it was for Jenn. It was a cure for the depressing and sullen aspects of Jenn's injury that needed a heavy infusion of levity for us to carry on and give her a happy, joyful life.

As Jenn's parent, I was totally focused on fixing her. That was important in the early stages of her recovery, but as time went on, I was relentless in looking for ways to get back the Jenn I knew prior to her injury. But Chris, Suzanne, and their families fully accepted the Jenn they knew post-accident.

"All my family think that Jenn is funny and happy just as she is," said Chris.

"Mine too," Suzanne added. "We can't think of her being any other way."

With no dark side from the past to inhibit their point of view, they freely allowed humor to drive their interactions with her, while our family viewed what happened to Jenn and her behaviors as tragic. To Chris and Suzanne, Jenn was not broken, and they were not focused on fixing her. Instead, they offered us the lesson of acceptance that our family would slowly understand and embrace.

Chapter 10

EATING ISSUES

TBI survivors often have a problem with self-initiation—they might be very thirsty but have no clue what to do about it. When Jenn first started going to the refrigerator, getting out a container of milk or juice, and getting herself a drink, it was viewed as a very positive sign and was amazing to witness. But what seemed to be a great step forward early in recovery soon became a problem to manage.

There didn't appear to be a signal between Jenn's gut and her brain telling her that she was full and to stop eating or drinking. Because of the caloric intake from her newfound skill, weight became yet another concern. Being overweight would add more medical issues to her condition. We needed to stop the conveyor belt of food going into her mouth.

Jenn was sneaky and determined to consume as much food as she could. Consistently watching her and keeping food out of her reach was only one aspect of managing this problem.

State regulatory agencies made frequent, mandated visits to the group homes overseeing the care of clients. One of their items of concern would be staff stopping a client from getting food if they wanted it. State guidelines dictated that this was a client's right. They were allowed to consume food when they desired it unless they were deemed medically unable to do so.

This regulation posed a problem when it came to Jennifer. I respected the state's interest in preserving the rights of clients, but it was an unhealthy and unrealistic ruling as it pertained to my daughter. While representatives were at Squire, food was not left out for easy taking. Everything was carefully put away, which served as the first deterrent for Jenn. If she did happen to get something, we had to let her have it during the inspection. Taking Jenn out of the house during those inspections was our best line of defense and the most effective.

Jenn's memory was long when it came to anything involving food. We didn't doubt that, in no time at all, she would connect the state's visits with a free-for-all to take whatever goodies she wanted.

But the state was only a small link in the chain of dealing with Jenn's obsession with food. The biggest one was that everyone loved to feed her!

Giving Jenn little tastes or bites of food was rewarding because she would shower the person with smiles, laughs, and arm squeezes, showing how much she appreciated any morsel they would share. No one could sit down and eat without having her hanging close by begging for a handout. She would position herself right at someone's elbow with an outstretched open hand, waiting for them to give her something. If you didn't offer anything, she would get upset and cry and whine. Of course, one bite was never enough—she wanted more. Each tidbit was quickly popped into her mouth, and within seconds her hand was out for the next piece.

One little bite was not a bad thing for Jenn, but this pattern continued throughout the day, every day, with all the staff or visitors that came to the group home. Someone was always eating in the house, and Jenn always wanted her share.

Soon the pounds started to add up. I coached the staff about not giving Jenn snacks, but it was a losing battle. Even Chris and Suzanne's kids loved sharing their goodies with Aunt Jenn—she appreciated it so much.

Finally, I took the extreme measure of putting Jenn on a diet plan and making everyone document any food she ate. As a team, the girls and I decided to go with the Weight Watchers program since many in the house were familiar with its guidelines, and it gave a clear-cut method of documenting food intake. The real beauty was that the plan offered food options for Jenn that were considered "free," meaning that you could eat as much of it as you wanted without gaining weight. One free food was plain popcorn. Other things included cut up vegetables like carrots, peppers, and celery.

Once implemented, the Weight Watchers program worked beautifully. It wasn't really Jenn that we were controlling, it was the people around her. All the staff were on board to help us keep a handle on Jenn's weight. If they were having a snack, they would hand Jenn some popcorn, a couple of kernels at a time, and she seemed as satisfied as if they'd given her their french fries or other high-calorie thing they were eating.

Chris and Suzanne's kids adjusted to the plan. If they were having a snack, they made sure they had something on the diet to hand to her. Jenn was happy, and one more hurdle was out of the way.

But as quickly as one problem was solved, a new one would arise. There was never a pause button in my oversight of Jenn's life. No matter how long it had been since the accident or how much progress she made, I would mostly notice all the things that had yet to be corrected and didn't allow myself to appreciate the accomplishments I'd made. My mind was always pondering solutions to perceived faults in my programs, or ways we were handling situations that could be improved. There was so much more that needed fixing, and I couldn't let it go. I always tried to move Jenn's recovery along, to push her forward and give her every opportunity to flourish. That was my job, and my life's work.

Chapter 11

THE OFFICE

Everything about the group home at Squire Court proved to be the perfect placement for Jenn, but I saw one problem. It was hard to escape the countless distractions that competed for her attention when I wanted to work on developing her cognitive skills.

Although Jenn and I worked on developing her skills in the sitting room at the back of the house, the kitchen with its tantalizing aromas and sounds would catch her focus better than the information I tried to present to her. We could hear the front door opening and closing as people came and went. Voices of staff, fellow housemates, or the television created a din that would break my concentration as well as Jenn's, even though we were as far removed as possible from it all. None of this was conducive to having a quiet place to work with Jenn on the communication skills that I considered important. We needed a quiet place where we could have structure and storage for the materials used in Jenn's learning programs.

I began searching for a small office space, keeping in mind price, size, and location. A simple room would do, but it needed to be close to Squire for easy access. I found a great choice beneath the Peacock Alley Mall in Danbury. It was spacious, inexpensive, and only ten minutes away from Squire. What more could I ask for? I signed the lease and was ready to introduce Jenn to her new learning space.

There were no furnishings or decorative touches on the ground floor entrance to the office area that was housed below the mall, only a glass encased directory of the businesses located there. JENN'S OFFICE was listed as one of them. It was an odd but nice feeling to see those words posted in black and white.

Once we entered the lower level, there was a small circular garden with a lamp post and some fake plantings, giving it the look of a miniature park. To the left and right was a long corridor with various businesses on either side.

"This looks like Munchkinland," Chris proclaimed as she took in the scenery on her first visit to the office. There was a sense of magical, mystical surrealness about this place. My mind told me I was underground, but my eyes told me I was outside facing a line of storefronts with colorful window displays all along a welcoming walkway.

We walked halfway down the left corridor to Jenn's office. I unlocked the bright red door, and when I turned on the lights, the pale-yellow walls gave off a soft glow as though it were a sunny day. The office measured twelve by twenty-four feet and was separated into two areas. An L-shaped teak desk faced the window and held a computer monitor.

The soft cream, blue, and green window treatment I made gave just the right touch of warmth and professionalism for our office to fit in with other businesses in that wing of the corridor.

As Jenn stepped inside the doorway, she walked past the carefully selected prints hanging on the walls. The one to the left of the door was a street scene in Paris of a restaurant with a palette of warm hues in the color scheme of the office's curtains and walls. Its empty tables awaited patrons to come and enjoy an afternoon cup of tea or sweet cakes. The other print hanging on the wall opposite the window was a still life of green apples arranged on a tabletop. I reasoned that since this was Jenn's office, food needed to be the theme for the decor. The staff would recognize the significance of my choices even if Jenn didn't. In fact, nothing seemed to catch Jenn's eye. She ignored it all and headed to the back room.

I looked to Jenn for clues of how she perceived the surroundings. She was smiling and laughing as she walked in and made a quick scan of the first room, no doubt looking to see where the kitchen was. But after finding nothing like that, she went to check out the back area. In the corner was a small compact refrigerator. She peered inside—bottled water, boring! She closed the door and continued to explore this curious place we'd brought her to. She tried the handles on the two metal cabinets where I had stored records, but they were locked, so she moved to the black bookcases. Here were familiar items like crayons, colorful paper, scissors, Post-it Notes, a box (a replacement ink cartridge for the printer that when shaken didn't reveal any important information), and tape. Jenn picked up the tape, looked at us, and gave it an enthusiastic shake along with a grin and mischievous expression as though to say, "Any taping jobs needing to be done?"

Baskets on the shelves contained yarn, fabric, beads, string, wire, and small packets of stickers. Gingerly she picked up each item; some she brought to her nose and smelled, others she turned over and over as though she couldn't understand why they were there. Some, like yarn or index cards, were quickly put back. She had no way of knowing that the supplies she was checking out were the materials for her programs.

The office was small, but tasteful and inviting. I was comfortable there and hoped the girls and Jenn shared my feelings.

WE WERE NO longer in charted territory as we began searching for methods to help Jenn reach new heights of accomplishment. All the educational programs were developed as a team effort by Chris, Suzanne, Amy, Mark, and me. Amy was an invaluable resource as she was in graduate school studying to be a speech–language pathologist.

Materials and equipment were in place, and the one-hour sessions were carefully laid out with formal descriptions, goals, and methods. Tracking of progress was documented with charts and graphs. Reports were prepared from this data and were included in the quarterly review sessions Ability held for each of their clients.

To help Jenn with communication and other cognitive issues, we needed to know what memories she'd retained after her accident. What skills were trapped in her brain that she had trouble accessing. We had to help her tap into those memories if they existed or develop new pathways of learning if they didn't. This was not a tried-and-true approach to treatment but rather a trial-and-error plan we designed specifically for her.

It was particularly important for Jenn to have a way to communicate. Body language was only effective to a point. I was determined to find a way to access some other method that would work for her.

Could Jenn understand the meaning behind photographs and pictures? Could we teach her to understand images? Was there another way of communicating with her: sign language, computer systems, pictures or written words that would open the door for us to access Jenn's thoughts and ideas, and let her know what we were trying to tell her?

Amy thought that possibly Amerind—American Indian gestures—would work.

"Mom, these hand and body movements aren't language based. Instead, they resemble the gestures we would use if we were trying to communicate with a person from a foreign country. If we wanted food, we might bring our fingers to our mouth and then do the chewing movement. This usually gets the other person to point in a particular direction indicating which way to go for food."

That sounded like a possibility for Jenn. A program was orchestrated where we'd say the word "eat," take a single Goldfish cracker in our fingers, and bring it to our mouth. Chris showed Jenn how to make the "eat" gesture and rewarded her by handing her a cracker when she copied it. Excitement over the bag of Goldfish treats had Jenn's body practically pulsing with electrical energy. She couldn't sit still. It was as though a million mosquitos were nibbling at her skin, and she had to move to stop the itch.

Frantic to get the Goldfish snacks, Jenn made sloppy attempts at the gesture and quickly offered her hand for the reward. Many times during the session, it seemed that Jenn could understand what the movement meant as she would get really excited when we did the "eat" gesture. In later sessions when we brought the snack out, she got excited but didn't spontaneously make the appropriate gesture. She didn't display a clear pattern of carrying through with the program.

As so often happened with Jenn, just when you thought she understood something, the next time she was clueless about it. After many weeks of practice, that particular experiment in communication didn't produce the outcome we'd hoped for, so we abandoned it.

At the office, I always sat to the side to let either Chris or Suzanne conduct the session. As the observer, I studied all the interactions between Jenn and her teacher. How did she perform on a task, was she engaged or bored? I looked for clues for what to try next and how to break the steps of a task down further into more manageable pieces.

When one method of communication failed, we attempted another. I dreamed up the idea of an activity board that displayed objects representing what Jenn was going to be working on that day. We attached Velcro to the back of things like keys, a pen, a miniature shoe, and a computer mouse and stuck them on the felt board. As I watched Suzanne place the activity board on the desk in front of Jenn, I was more confident about this approach than I had been with some of our past efforts.

"Jenn, let's work on the computer," Suzanne said as she pointed to the real computer mouse and the miniature one hanging on the board.

"Give me the mouse, Jenn, so we can work on the computer."

Jenn smiled and giggled but didn't seem to understand the words or gestures. It might take weeks of training to make a breakthrough. I didn't expect her to grasp the concept during that first session, but I thought this method of communication had potential.

After months of practice had passed, she did learn to remove one of the objects or pictures from the activity board when we pointed to an activity such as the computer or a pen. The problem was that her selection didn't match the task that was being shown to her by Chris or Suzanne.

We tried a different approach. We let Jenn pick one object from the board to see if she would initiate the next step of reaching for the task that it represented. That too met with failure. I also noticed that her choices were random—she didn't pick objects in order of her favorite tasks such as taping or stapling.

Jenn never exhibited the ability to associate the task she was going to work on with the object she removed from the board. Why would she fail so miserably at this program when she clearly understood things outside the office like the connection between car keys and going for a ride in her car? To get Jenn excited about leaving Squire, the girls just showed her those keys. She also understood when you showed her a dinner plate that she was about to get food. Why did she understand some connections but not others? This was another unanswered question for the long list that ran through my mind since the accident.

ONE OF JENN'S computer activities involved using index cards, each with an individual word printed on it. When we showed it to her, we'd hold up a picture of what was written on the card and direct her to type the word into the computer.

It took many weeks of practice, but eventually Jenn became familiar with the placement of individual letters on the keyboard and could quickly type what she saw on the index cards.

"Jenn, type 'Mom,'" Chris said, showing her the card and photo. Dutifully, Jenn typed in the correct letters and then seemed to look to Chris for reassurance that she had completed the task successfully.

"Good job, Jenn. Do it again," Chris said pointing at the keyboard.

Jenn repeated her task with total compliance; her smile indicated to me that she was pleased with herself for getting such positive feedback from Chris.

Once adept at typing each word, we took away one element of the drill. Chris just showed Jenn the picture of me.

"Who's this, Jenn, can you type this word?" Jenn giggled, looked at Chris, then at the photo, but did nothing with the keyboard, even when Chris gestured toward it.

Over the course of many weeks, try as we might to have Jenn show us she could translate a photo into a typed word, it didn't happen. Instead, she'd perseverate on one particular letter key, any letter, repeatedly tapping it over and over again, unable to duplicate any of the words she had previously typed when shown an index card.

Disappointment rang loudly in my head. I had placed a lot of hope on pictures giving us a pathway to communicate with Jenn, but as before, we had no positive results.

Computer preschool learning games that focused on matching items were also techniques that we tried. Again, Jenn was not able to understand or define the meaning of the images she was seeing. Unfortunately, all attempts at having her recognize pictures as a means of language failed.

I thought that if we connected her memory to a time before computers, we might have a breakthrough—pen and paper came to mind. She could use these tools, but she just scribbled lines across the paper. We drew pictures to see if she would follow our example. Other than occasionally copying a few basic shapes that we'd drawn, squares or circles, this idea also dead-ended.

As another exercise in using pens and paper, we set

a goal of getting Jenn to write her name. This wasn't as much about communicating as it was curiosity on my part to see if she could do it. After several weeks of coaching, she established a script rhythm and could smoothly write the *e* and *nn* after someone helped with the first letter, *J*. The *J* was the missing piece of her memory that stopped her from fully writing her first name. We had her repeat the motion of writing the *J* for many weeks, and slowly the entire word began to flow out in a natural way. At last, Jenn had a signature—a messy one, but we didn't care. That signature would grace all future special occasion cards that Jenn gave out to family and friends. She also used this signature to sign the attendance sheets at her quarterly meetings at Ability. I don't know if she understood that this was her name or signature, but she was aware that it made all of us happy when she did it, and we knew that she loved pleasing us.

Curiously, during the time we were pushing to help Jenn with language, I asked Chris and Suzanne what their kids thought about Jenn's lack of communication. Their answers surprised me.

"Our kids think she understands everything," both Chris and Suzanne told me on more than one occasion.

All the Boisvert and Benz kids knew Aunt Jenn didn't talk but felt that she clearly knew what was going on. I knew her way of connecting with people with body language was extraordinary, but for these young people to believe that Aunt Jenn was totally tuned into the things going on around her was bewildering to me.

Yes, her vivid facial expressions and gestures spoke volumes about how she was responding to any given situation. She could be flirtatious, cunning, curious, ecstatic, and furious—and she was very clear in expressing those feelings. She did seem to quickly read the feelings and emotions of others, and often reacted accordingly. Body language was the only method she had to engage people, and it was obvious that connecting with others was important to her—she actively pursued anyone nearby who might give her attention. She wanted that human contact and worked effectively to develop the only means available to her—body language. In reflecting back on this, I recognize that she understood her limitations more than I did. Jenn was the one who, on her own, developed an effective system of communication with others that worked.

NOT ONLY DID we work on cognitive skills at Jenn's office, we also endeavored to improve the physical function of her injured hand. As a right-handed person pre-accident, having limited use of it was another challenge for her, and quickly she began the process of making herself left-hand dominant. Although adept at using her left hand in many daily tasks, for things that required more dexterity or the use of two hands working together, Jenn would become greatly frustrated. Left to her own devices, she would just choose to skip doing any two-handed task such as buttoning a shirt or zipping up her coat.

With the right side of Jenn's body compromised by her TBI, her right hand and elbow had very limited movement. The finger that had been surgically repaired had limited range of motion, but the rest of that hand was also compromised. It was stiff, and she always held it in a fisted position. She used it more as a weight to hold things down than as a grasping tool for fine motor function.

At the office, various programs were devised for Jenn

to use her right hand for things like the typing exercise we had her work on at each session. We also brought in several articles of clothing for her to practice manipulating zippers and buttons with both hands working together on the task.

Jenn seemed to totally ignore her whole right arm. Her brain appeared to have a hard time recognizing that she had that appendage. Throughout the day, we were constantly cueing her to bring her arm and hand into action instead of holding it motionless and close to her chest as she was prone to do. Occupational therapy continued at Ability, and with their guidance, we pushed her to use that hand to maintain the little remaining function she had with it.

I got the idea that working at the office on simple tasks such as writing, cutting paper, or putting beads on a piece of yarn would stimulate both her cognitive function and the use of her right arm and hand.

When I had the girls start teaching Jenn how to tie shoes, it was a task specifically designed to employ her right hand. Although reluctant to use that hand at first, she knew we expected this from her and tried to comply, but she seemed to have no clue how to start.

Chris and Jenn purchased a cute pair of pink sneakers the day before we started this new skill program. I loved their choice of something fun and girly for this project. Chris began doing hand-over-hand crossing of the laces with her, the first step in the process of making a bow. It was wonderful that Jenn had become less resistant to this kind of touching. I had a flashback to early times when that kind of contact would have sent her into a fit of rage. Now, she was not only compliant, but she seemed to enjoy the interaction during the office sessions. As I watched, she giggled, had a big toothy smile on her face, and gave Chris an arm squeeze.

Within just a few sessions, I saw that Jenn knew the next steps: making the loops and bringing them together in the tie. An old memory had popped to the surface and allowed her to complete the shoe-tying process.

Repeated work over several weeks helped her learn how to initiate the one missing piece of how to tie her shoes—crossing the laces. Was it worth all the effort to do something that could so easily be done for her? Without question–*yes*! The value was that she had learned a new skill, tapped into her memory, and used two hands together on a task. I was ecstatic; the gears in my brain began spinning. What else could I help Jenn recover from the past? Were most of her disabilities a single step away from evaporating if I found the missing link in her brain that would connect the pieces?

The shoelace project had opened my eyes, and I was on a roll to evaluate other daily living skills that she was not yet able to do. I decided to break each task down into the different steps required for completion to see which parts she knew, and which ones had to be relearned. She had adapted to her new post-accident world in some rather profound ways. Now I had to figure out how to give her the tools she needed to make even more skills available to her.

EVER SO PATIENT and lighthearted, Chris and Suzanne used the office time effectively, but they had to keep the momentum going with a lot of "what if?" trial-and-error programs. Never shy about trying something different, they offered more than their share of ideas. They made the office a fun experience for Jenn, so she was always encouraged with positive feedback, regardless of how slow or inaccurate her performance was.

The girls said, "What if Jenn helped take care of someone else, like a child. Would that bring out some different aspects of her personality?" Starting with a baby doll in the office, Jenn was instructed on how to dress and undress the doll. This was good therapy for her two hands, but would it result in any other positive outcome?

Christine decided to bring the idea home and have Jenn help bathe Lily, her youngest child, who was just two years old. Lily was game. She loved Aunt Jenn, and it was another way to interact with one of her favorite people. With video camera in hand, Chris was ready to record the whole episode for me.

The bath water was already drawn, and Lily was excitedly splashing around in the tub, waiting for Aunt Jenn to begin the process of washing her. Jenn was hanging back, watching Lily. She seemed to think that she was only going to be the observer, not the doer.

"Go ahead Jenn, start washing Lily," Chris encouraged as she handed Jenn the washcloth.

Jenn gave a halfhearted laugh and shook the washcloth at Chris before trying to hand it back.

"No Jenn, you do it. Wash Lily."

Chris placed a small stool next to the tub, and helped Jenn lower herself down for easy access.

With their volume set on high, Jenn and Lily laughed, ramping up for what they must have thought was going to be a pretty funny experience. Washcloth in hand, Jenn started with a few scrubbing motions on Lily's belly which made both of them crack up even more. The noise in the small bathroom resonated at a near deafening level, but no one cared—Lily and Jenn were having fun.

Watching the video, I was surprised to see how gentle Jenn was as she washed Lily. When she was excited or grumpy, her actions were usually rough and far from the careful, motherly way in which she was carrying out this new bathing task. This was my first lesson learned from the video: Jenn understood the importance of being gentle with Lily. She could be laughing uproariously and still maintain enough control of herself to use a soothing touch when approaching a small child.

"Do more, Jenn. Wash Lily's legs," Chris said as she pointed to Lily's lower body. Lily was standing in the tub, making it easier for Jenn who ran the washcloth down one leg and then the other, but only the front, ignoring the back of her legs.

"Now wash here," Chris directed, pointing to Lily's back. With encouragement, Jenn lovingly complied and even gave a quick dab on the back of Lily's legs.

Lily continued to splash around the tub, enjoying the rush small kids seem to get as they feel the warm liquid run off their skin and see the trickles of water slide down the tiles. And Lily's excitement generated a similar reaction from Jenn as the two of them interacted without words, but with laughter and visual expressions of pure joy that come with the wonders of bath time.

But the water was cooling down, and it was time for Lily to hop out of the tub so Jenn could begin drying her off.

"Okay Lily, time to get out." And as quickly as the words were out of Chris's mouth, Lily climbed over the edge of the bathtub which for her was a high hurdle.

Chris picked up the towel, handed it to Jenn, and pointed to Lily. Jenn seemed to understand what she was supposed to do next. She gently supported Lily with her bad arm as she dried her with the other. It wasn't a thorough job, but she did it gently and lovingly. Tears welled up in my eyes as I watched the video of Jenn perform her task with such cautious care and compassion. Feelings of love and warmth flooded me as though a summer's breeze had brushed against my skin, leaving me touched by the gentle wonder of it. My daughter had just shown me a deeper side of her new, complex, and compromised self. She understood so much more than I had given her credit for.

Chris handed Jenn the pajama bottoms and said, "Help Lily get dressed."

I knew that Jenn didn't always know where different pieces of clothing were supposed to go. Early in her recovery, clothing was as foreign to her as any of the other things she was introduced to. Once she learned that clothing belonged on the body, Jenn was as likely to put her legs into the sleeves of a shirt or her arms in the legs of her pants as she was to stick her head in either the sleeve or leg. But she had come a long way from those days.

She carefully held the pajamas open at the waist for Lily to step into. The bottoms were going on backward, but neither Jenn nor Lily knew that. Chris then handed her the top. Jenn inspected it, as if to determine exactly how she was going to get Lily into it and then, using both hands, held it open for Lily to stick her head through. After Lily had her arms in both sleeves, Jenn helped adjust the garment, so all was perfect, and Lily was dressed.

Jenn had taken the information she used each day to bathe and dress herself and applied it to someone else. This was a big deal. It was the kind of step that doesn't come naturally to a person who has suffered a severe head injury. They are often not able to take the information learned in one setting and apply it elsewhere. In the video, I saw that Jenn had carried learned skills into another situation, revealing a much higher level of cognition that encouraged me to look for even more ways to have her utilize her abilities.

FROM TIME TO time, I saw the need to have a pow-wow with the staff to go over new materials or programs. Jenn's office was the perfect quiet meeting place for us, while Bagelman, our favorite lunch spot, served as our unofficial meeting place for less formal discussions.

The purpose of these meetings was to explore new ideas and develop programs that looked promising. Once discussed, we had to prepare all the documentation to outline the goals of these programs and how we were going to track Jenn's performance. Ability trained their staff to be well versed in documentation, so Chris and Suzanne knew exactly how each idea would translate into a formal program for Jenn.

Jenn always sat in on our discussions. She was very animated and would act as if she were taking part in the conversations. During these meetings, Jenn would sometimes maneuver to get right in front of the face of the person closest to her to get some personal attention. This brief exchange seemed to be a way for her to acknowledge that she was there and listening. She had no visual feedback from us on what was being discussed that would help her to understand the meaning of our words. All that she knew was that her people were gathered around the table having a discussion, and she seemed more than happy to share in the experience.

A favorite pastime for Jenn, when not actively engaged in something, was *picking*. Picking a hole in the finish of wooden furniture, picking a hole in her sweater and pulling a loose thread out, picking at the upholstery on the sofa or leather seat of the car—most any object would suffice to satisfy this compulsion. Her sweaters and shirts were prime targets, especially because they were always readily available. I was never given a professional opinion on the reason for

Jenn's picking activity, but it seemed to fall in line with other odd behaviors she took on after her injury.

While sitting through the meetings at her office, she had time on her hands to pick, and she had a favorite spot on the desk she worked on. Once she had the hole started, she would work to increase the size, removing flecks of varnish and brushing them aside to clean the area. Another piece of furniture was branded with Jenn's special insignia.

One of the programs we developed at the office and took out into the community was photography. Before her accident, Jenn, inspired by her father's love of this hobby, had loved taking photos. If she were equipped with a decent camera, we wanted to see if she still had any memories of how to take snapshots. It would be a great way to have her coordinate using both her hands.

I put the camera strap around her neck and handed her the camera.

"Jenn, take a picture of Suzanne," I prompted as I pointed to Suzanne.

She held it up close to her face, not directly to her eye, then tilted it down to see where the button was to take the shot. She demonstrated that she remembered the concept of taking pictures, but the mechanics of it were troublesome. Even with repeated tries, the awkward use of her right hand caused her to either point the lens up at the ceiling or down on the floor. We continued the program for several weeks but, encountering little success, moved on to other things.

Just because Jenn couldn't effectively use the camera didn't mean it would go to waste.

On my next visit to Squire, Chris told me about the latest fun thing she and Jenn had done.

"I decided to do a photo shoot of Jenn on Tuesday. It was a beautiful fall day, and the foliage was in full color. I wanted to spend as much time outside as we could before the doldrums of winter set in, so I drove to the park in Bethel to take some pictures.

"Jenn seemed a little confused at first about why we were there, but as I worked with her on how to pose for me, she really got into the idea.

"Look at these shots, Barb. Jenn was so agreeable and didn't try to leave or anything. She seemed to know what we were doing and was having a lot of fun hamming it up for me and the camera."

I was stunned at the beautiful photos Chris showed me. Jenn was in her stylish black leather jacket, and her hair was in a classy updo; she looked every bit the part of a model. Chris always had a good eye for composition, but the shots taken that day looked professional. Our favorite was Jenn posing as she leaned against a tree. Appropriately framed today as an eight-by-ten, this picture remains a treasured image of our daughter—happy and having a fun day with one of her best friends.

BOTH CHRIS AND Suzanne loved to test Jenn's memory when they drove her to our house in Washingtonville. Once the girls exited off Interstate 84 and were within five miles of their destination, Jenn would become very excitable and loud. It was clear to the driver that she knew she was going home. To test this theory, they would sometimes intentionally turn the wrong way, and sure enough, Jenn would become agitated and angry at their error.

Jenn knew, from the first time we brought her home after the accident, the layout of our house and exactly where her bedroom was. As soon as she walked in the door, she unhesitatingly turned left down the hallway and went straight into her room.

One time the wall phone rang in the kitchen, and Jenn tried to answer it. But then she stopped, had a puzzled look on her face, and seemed to realize that she either didn't know what to do next or didn't have the language to proceed any further. At that point, with a somewhat confused smile on her face, she handed the phone to her dad.

If Jenn could remember her way home and everything about our house, did she remember other places around Washingtonville? Frequently, we'd take her on a drive around the town, passing where she'd worked and gone to school. We also drove by her friends' houses, local malls, and stores. She never showed us that any of these buildings had significance to her, as she made no verbalizations or emotional display of recognition. Only our house stimulated those responses.

SPECULATING AND THEORIZING about what Jenn did and didn't know was an ongoing topic of conversation between her staff and our family. We could never figure her out or find all the answers to our questions. Jenn was complex and mystifying and always had us guessing about what was going on in her head. But we were all united in wanting to discover what she could do and how much she could learn, and we loved exploring Jenn's mindset and her surprising abilities.

Chapter 12

MEDICAL PUZZLE

There was a medical mystery regarding Jenn's language ability. The assessment that she had no language after her injury was not entirely true. Strange occurrences of vocalization did happen at times, but not often, and not with any regularity. Each time they happened was a surprise—a nice one.

While Jenn was at the first rehab facility, she said many words that were intertwined with her moaning and mutterings. In September of 1991, just two months after her accident, she was vocalizing more and more each day, which was encouraging to us and to the professionals working with her. Jenn spoke Amy's name several times and offered Greg's name when someone asked who her boyfriend was. Greg was a regular visitor, and the staff knew his relationship to Jenn. Occasionally we got some appropriate "yes" and "no" answers to questions and when asked about her arm, she would reply, "It hurts," or "I'm fine."

Jenn often mumbled threatening phrases to the occupational therapist who regularly had to stretch her injured right hand and arm. "I'm gonna hurt ya," was something Jenn often said because there was no doubt that what the therapist was doing was painful, and she wanted her to stop. And anyone who Jenn felt was bothering her might get an "f-you" response.

She spent many weeks after her accident powerless to ward people off, but now with her increased strength, she was lashing out. Everyone around her had to be careful, as this was the more agitated phase of her recovery when she would not only mumble obscenities at you but, given the chance, would bite you as well. Similar to other phases in her recovery, this aggressive state didn't last too long.

When Jenn talked during those first few months at Hillcrest, it was not conversational. Her verbalizations were an occasional word or phrase: "I leave here" or "I afraid." Her use of singular words or brief phrases continued for about six months. And then they stopped.

No amount of coaching or encouragement would prompt Jenn to utter any words. Sometimes her mouth would move as if she were speaking, but no sound would come out. Other times, she uttered random syllables. In place of words, Jenn screeched, screamed, and had a piercing whine and groan. None of us knew why she stopped progressing with her language skills.

In the fall of 1992, many months after her last words were spoken, Jenn surprised us while at home for the weekend. It was a Sunday, so the whole family went to the local outlet stores at Woodbury Commons. Amy needed a homecoming dress, and it was a beautiful day to stroll through the shops in the open-air mall. Purchases in hand, we headed through the parking lot to the car. Partway there Jenn announced, "I want to eat more."

That stopped us dead in our tracks! "What did you say, Jenn?"

She carefully repeated, "I want to eat more."

Okay! We immediately headed to a nearby restaurant and promised her anything she asked for. Although she didn't utter any additional words, we ordered dinner for all of us and spent a lovely time sharing a meal together.

A couple of days later around lunchtime at Hillcrest, Jenn said, "I want to eat some." Everyone jumped at the chance to reinforce her newly found communication skills by quickly bringing out a tasty meal for her. She must have enjoyed the food as she quickly consumed everything on her plate. We hoped that the immediate reward of giving her food at her request would encourage more words, but that didn't happen—the talking stopped again. No one could tell us why. I did a lot of research on brain injury and aphasia but found nothing that resembled the on-again, off-again speech pattern Jenn exhibited.

I was excited and encouraged when Jenn talked, especially when she was able to express herself clearly. I had hoped that, by this time, her speech would develop into true communication. For us, it was devastating each time her speech came to a halt. This was not willful on Jenn's part—we could tell she wanted to communicate. She looked right at us when she wanted to say something and would mouth noises with facial expressions, but no words came out. Something in her brain must have blocked her from accessing her language center. Over the next year, Jenn was unable to say any more words.

ON SEPTEMBER 7, 1993, two years after the accident, Jenn had her first seizure. She was living at Squire and was taken to Danbury Hospital where blood tests and a CAT scan were performed, confirming that she'd had a seizure. After monitoring her overnight and seeing that she presented no new medical issues, she returned to the group home.

Seizures are common after a head injury, but we were still surprised because, for the two years since her accident, she'd had none. Doctors had put her on anti-seizure meds right after her injury, but after a year and a half of no seizure activity, she was taken off the drug. Anti-seizure meds can hamper cognition, and we wanted to give her every possible advantage to progress in her recovery.

Two days after her seizure, we received an excited call from the staff at Squire Court. "You have to come; Jenn is talking!" We couldn't get there fast enough.

When we walked in the door of Squire, Jenn happily walked right up to us, gave us a hug, and said, "My parents." Those words were monumental. We stood there, barely able to take this in. Until that moment, we were not sure if she knew who we were. It was possible that to her we were just the nice people who came on a regular basis and took her out to eat. Now we knew that Jenn recognized us as her family.

Mark and I could hardly contain our excitement and were desperate to engage her in conversation.

"Jenn, it is so good to hear you talk again. We've missed your words—tell us more," I encouraged. She smiled and giggled a couple of times before turning to her dad and giving his arm a squeeze.

"What can you tell us, Jenn?" Mark asked, but other than a giggle, she didn't give a direct answer. Mark had a video camera in hand and was ready to capture any remarks she might give. When he pointed it at her, it prompted this response.

"It's funny," she said, giggling.

"What's funny, Jenn?" he asked. She turned in my direction to again comment, "It's funny."

"Jenn, can you say a few more words for me?" Mark tried again but got no response.

Chris suggested, "Try offering her this pretzel and see if she will say anything."

Sure enough, Jenn's eyes beamed with excitement as Mark held out the treat.

"It's Jennifer Ann's," she said in a very soft voice. We could barely make out the "Jennifer Ann's" part of her remark.

"What did you say, Jenn. Tell me again," Mark implored.

"It's Jennifer Ann's," she repeated.

Interesting that Jenn was saying her first and middle name. As she was growing up, I would say, "Jennifer Ann" when I was upset or angry with her. Both my girls thought it was funny that I called them different names when I really wanted their attention—for Amy, it was Amy Rubin, and for Jenn it was Jennifer Ann. I guess that by using two words in their names, I thought it would have greater impact. Neither girl referred to themselves that way, so it was very curious that Jenn was doing it now.

Mark and I were glued to each and every word Jenn said. The house staff was equally engaged in trying to get her to talk by offering snacks or doing silly things to make her laugh or say something. All of us delighted in anything she said, even though most of her talking consisted of only about two or three repeated phrases.

We spent a blissful two hours with Jenn, but it was getting late and time for us to head home. It was always hard to leave Jenn at Squire after a visit, but it was particularly difficult that night. As we began to make our way to the door, she came over and gave us another hug and a goodbye kiss—the normal affection our pre-accident Jenn would have given us. Since her injury, we had only gotten halfhearted hugs and a movement of her face toward our cheek, giving us a slight bump on the face. She didn't seem to know how to purse her lips to form an actual kiss. That night her kiss was perfect and warmed my heart, giving me hope for further progress.

"Do you believe the difference in Jenn?" I asked Mark on our drive home. "I so want to keep this version. It was our best day since the accident."

I saw all the possibilities for her as my mind reeled with positive images that popped into my head. Life would return to normal, and Jenn would be able to live at home and go back to school. Happiness and pure joy pulsed through my body.

Mark was quick to add, "Not only was she calm, she acted more like our original Jenn."

"I know, it was like our pre-accident daughter was back," I agreed. The person we saw that night was the Jenn we knew so well and had missed over the past two years.

"I hate that I have to go to work tomorrow," Mark said. "I want to go back up to Squire and spend more time with her—it's so much like having our old Jenn back. And I agree, the difference in her whole personality was wonderful. I just hope it stays that way."

The hour's drive home was filled with speculation about where this improved level of communication and behavior was going to lead her. At that moment in time, we dared to see the future as bright and our life restored to its former self. It was a nice way to cap off a remarkable evening.

Sunday, three days after she began talking, we brought her home for the day. Walking up the sidewalk from the driveway to the front door, Jenn said, "It's wrong house." Since her accident, we had changed the exterior of the house from cedar shakes to medium tan vinyl siding. The house looked different, but we had brought Jenn home many times since her accident, so this proclamation surprised us. Was this the first time that she recognized the change, or was it just the first time she could verbalize the difference?

In the days that followed, our family and the staff tried to get Jenn to engage in conversation or answer the many questions we had. But try as we might, she seemed incapable of conversing in a normal manner. Only random words or phrases were spoken just like before, but we were nailed to every utterance. Staff took notes of the words she said during that time and captured more video of some brief moments of her talking. All this was done to document the medical breakthrough in her recovery.

A truly sad thing that Jenn repeated was the phrase, "The way I was." It was heartbreaking for us to think that she could see how she had changed. Had she known all along? Possibly this realization had become apparent to her only because, along with speech, she was thinking more clearly and could accurately assess the reality of her disabilities.

But even with Jenn talking, it was unclear if she understood what we were saying. As we spoke to her, something still didn't seem to connect.

As before, we were not having conversations with her during those exchanges. Instead, she was randomly saying a few simple phrases, often with the same repeated content. The loud, booming volume that had become her post-accident voice was replaced with an angelic, soft-spoken tone that exuded joy and happiness. There was always a bit of soft laughter resonating with each of her spoken words, a distant echo of our pre-accident Jenn.

But all our hopes for her newfound speech came to a crushing end. As each new day passed, her speech became less and less frequent until it vanished a week later. Along with the loss of talking, her personality reverted back to the loud and excitable person she had become since her injury. This was heartbreaking for everyone, especially Mark and me. When we saw those glimpses of our original Jennifer, we had dared to hope and let down our carefully constructed defense systems. When she reverted back to the post-accident Jenn, Mark and I had to comfort each other again for another loss. We fell hard, and as always, had no idea what the future would bring.

IN THE YEARS ahead, we would be able to look back and note an unusual pattern: Jenn experienced a medical event almost every autumn. September of 1991 brought the first talking experience she had. In the fall of 1992, over a year after her accident, she needed surgery to remove a section of her skull that became infected at the site of the initial brain surgery. A year later in 1993, she had the seizure and prolonged talking episode. In the fall of 1994, the missing piece of skull was replaced with a composite material, and the following year, in 1995, there was surgery on Jenn's right elbow to release the atrophied muscles and tendons with the goal of giving her more range of motion. Other fall events included gallbladder surgery and later three more grand mal seizures requiring hospitalization in 2007, 2008 and 2009.

Her intermittent talking also only made appearances in the fall, especially after a seizure or anesthesia from a surgery. We came to view this time of year with a lot of anticipation. What was it about the fall that triggered those events? Staff questioned if that was the season when she had her accident, but no—that had happened in the summer. The first autumn after her accident was when she emerged from the fog of her coma, but how would that have had an impact on future fall happenings? Professionals, friends, and family all theorized about these strange occurrences, but they remained a mystery.

Over the years, we were to see a repeat of Jenn's fragmented talking, but it was never for as long or as profound as in the fall of 1993. We can only guess that the damage in Jenn's brain left her with a very fragile connection to the language center, and the seizures might have increased brain activity in that region for a very limited time span, allowing her some access to language function. Perhaps anesthesia given during surgery stimulated the neurons in her brain in the same way her seizures did, because she would often talk shortly after a medical procedure.

Did this frustrate Jenn? To have the ability to talk and then have it gone would seem to be a devastating blow to anyone, but we didn't notice that reaction. Her lack of awareness was probably a good thing as she had no control over her speech skills, and it would not have served her well to know that she couldn't perform the same tasks as she had the previous day or even a few minutes before.

WHAT DID SHE see or hear? Jenn often stopped in the middle of a task, or when just sitting or standing, to look vacantly up or to the side in a frozen gaze. Always calm for those brief few seconds, she seemed content and blissful as she stared off into space. Chris and Suzanne referred to those times as when Jenn was seeing "pink elephants." Someone calling her name would always bring her back from wherever she was in those moments. She would make eye contact, but still seemed to not be totally engaged. These weird episodes passed within a minute, and once she was released from her stupor, Jenn's bubbly personality came roaring back, and she would excitedly continue with whatever she was doing as though nothing had happened.

We charted the staring episodes over several months and addressed the issue with two neurologists, but no conclusions were reached. Professionals thought that if Jenn responded to her name and looked at us, there wasn't cause for alarm.

What was it that called Jenn's attention to some unknown place? The calm she exhibited during those staring incidents resembled the times when she talked—was there a connection? The" look-aways," as we called them, did not start until after Jenn was living at Squire. Did something change in her brain that brought them on? Was this a harbinger of mental decay or a visual indication that new neuro pathways were connecting in her brain? There was no pattern to when the look-aways occurred, and there was never an association between them and the seizures that sometimes came in the fall. Their occurrence didn't change in frequency either before or after her seizures—they just were.

During a staring episode, Chris and Suzanne would jokingly ask Jenn if she was looking at those pink elephants again. She might give them a nod in response, even as her daze persisted for several more seconds. Was the nod confirming that she heard their voices, but she hadn't yet returned from her faraway place?

Jenn was a puzzle to me and all the professionals who worked with her. She kept us guessing, questioning, and at a loss for what all was going on in her brain. I was challenged but determined to uncover the answers that were not easily found. We were always trying to understand Jenn—and what might help her. It was a difficult challenge, no matter how much practice we had at doing it, but I for one could not simply accept what was—I wanted more.

Chapter 13

THE COURT AND
NEW YORK STATE

During all the goings-on in Jenn's post-accident life, there was another undercurrent, a constant player in the background that kept all of us on our toes and sometimes on edge. After winning the lawsuit, I still had to jump through a never-ending barrage of hoops to satisfy the court system.

I thought our court battles were over once the lawsuit was settled. Wrong! Family courts are responsible for oversight of the trust funds they have under their jurisdiction, and Jenn's trust fell within those parameters. Money was not awarded to a trust, never to be revisited by the court system. Guidelines for how the monies were to be administered and distributed were carefully laid out in volumes of legalese. Because the supplemental needs trust was new, it required even more legal review to fully understand the various aspects of its directives. States, courts, and individual law firms were challenged to interpret this new law and help clients meet its requirements, and I was caught in the middle of it all.

My business degree and experience in accounting helped me to secure the position as cotrustee along with the Bank of New York. I knew this was a rare privilege that I was awarded by the court, and it would prove to be an invaluable tool to help me to do my job of overseeing Jenn's affairs more smoothly. If a banking official had been awarded my position, it would have been a detriment to Jenn as they would have had little knowledge of the daily workings of our programs and would not have had a personal stake in their client's outcome.

It was a no-brainer that the bank should manage the investing aspects of the trust. They had the resources and expertise to handle that part of the account. My role was to manage the disbursements and prepare the spreadsheets to account for the monies spent. I opened a checking account to take care of smaller purchases and bills. Large expenditures, such as cars and quarterly payments to Ability Beyond Disability for staff, were done directly from the trust.

Each month I sent my spreadsheets to the bank outlining every expenditure made. The credit card statements provided a detailed itemization of most purchases. Squire provided the listings of purchases done with the small petty cash fund held for each client along with a receipt as documentation. The petty cash would be used to buy small items, like a package of gum or a soft drink.

By law I was required to keep a receipt for every purchase: bridge tolls, candy bars, movie tickets, subway tickets, car washes, carnival rides—everything. I packaged all of the receipts into monthly and yearly containers to be stored *forever*. All of the records were subject to review by the court and the Medicaid division of New York State if they needed to verify any of Jenn's expenditures.

Annually, the bank and I were required to send a detailed report to the court outlining the investment holdings and all expenditures made on Jenn's behalf during that year. Reams of paper detailed every stock and bond sale or purchase, the income generated by them, and how it was invested. Every purchase, be it salary paid for personal staff or something as simple as a package of Goldfish crackers, was included. It was mind-boggling that anyone would actually sift through all this, especially a busy court system. But they did.

Two years after the trust was established and functioning, the bank and I received a summons to make an appearance over what they perceived as a questionable item in the disbursements. A lawyer was retained to represent my interests and those of the bank, paid for by the trust. If that pricy expense weren't bad enough, I soon found out that the court had also hired an attorney to represent them, and the most mind-blowing part of it was that the trust would be billed for all their hours too.

I was not one to anger easily, but my blood boiled when I heard about these wasteful expenses. Where was the justice in this needless assault on money set aside for Jennifer in her trust? I was fuming as I spoke over the phone with the soft-spoken but authoritative woman who would be representing the bank and me.

"I can't believe the court expects the trust to pay for their lawyer. How is this even possible?" I questioned her.

"It really is a routine thing that courts do. They have a clerk review the accountings, and if that person has any questions, they call in legal counsel to review the documents and present their findings at a court appearance."

"What do you think is going to happen?" I again asked as my anger was laced with concern.

"I think we will be fine; it's just a matter of answering their questions. This trust is new, so I think they are more inclined to check that everything is being done correctly," she said.

Her assurances did little to cool the fire that burned in my gut as I pondered what was happening. It was one thing for the trust to pay for our legal counsel, but I was beside myself that it also had to pay for the court's attorney. I knew this was going to be a costly and time-consuming process, and my patience with the system was at a breaking point, especially when I heard what the questionable item was that initiated all this nonsense.

The red flag in our accounting was the three-day Carnival cruise trip Jenn had been taken on by Maria and sister Amy. That trip proved to be a beautiful bonding experience for two sisters who had been separated by a horrific tragedy and left with few opportunities to be together and have fun. Our attorney was given a heads-up on the specific issue by the court's legal counsel, so we were well prepared to defend our position on that expenditure.

In my conversations with our attorney, I wanted her to understand how ludicrous I thought it was that they were questioning this expense and what was at stake if they ruled against us.

"If the court takes this stand on trip expenditures, they're discriminating against a person who is disabled. They are essentially saying that Jenn should not have the same pleasures and privileges of travel in life as do others in our society. Why shouldn't a person who is disabled be able go places and do things if they have the necessary funds? If the expense does nothing to jeopardize the future solvency of a trust, and the person gets great joy from taking those trips, they have the right to venture beyond local attractions the same as anyone else does."

"I agree with you, and will present this to the court," she reassured me.

The day of the court appearance finally came and once again Mark and I climbed the long steps leading up to the county court building. As we made our way through the dingy corridor, I had a sense of an ominous storm brewing, even if it was only in my head. My nerves were on edge as we timidly made our way to the doorway marked FAMILY COURT.

Jenn's bank trustee and our attorney greeted us with outstretched hands offering firm handshakes. Both ladies, properly attired in sleek business suits, were looking composed and professional. It was comforting that Mark and I were not going to face this challenge alone.

Once all were seated and the judge entered the room, the court's attorney opened the case and began her argument. Her blonde bobbed hair bounced back and forth as she spoke.

"This trip was just a good time for the staff when their client would have been just as happy to go to the local zoo," the bobbing head proclaimed with acid dripping from her voice. She glanced over in our direction and gave us a smug grin, looking sure of herself and condescending. "There is no need for these kinds of costly adventures."

Our attorney was ready. "No person who is disabled should be restricted in what they can do by a court's perceived bias, if they have the means to travel beyond their home area. This would in fact be a case of discrimination if the court rules that my client should not have taken that trip. The trust is amply funded to support such an expense; its future solvency is not in question because of this trip or any other trips in the

future. And for the record, my client doesn't like the zoo!"
she said to add a little zing to her defense.

The judge carefully listened to our argument and after
some thought apparently had a hard time disputing the
appearance of discrimination if he ruled against us. "Everything seems in order," he said. "Case dismissed!"

We left the court feeling victorious, but the thousands
of dollars in legal fees to reach that point had me livid. The
costs to attain that positive outcome far exceeded the expense
of the trip. In principle, I thought we had made a very clear
point with the court about discrimination, and I hoped it
would have a lasting impact. It did—until the next time.

Two years later, a new red flag came up and another
court appearance was scheduled because of a forty-dollar
purchase from a jewelry store. Seriously? A forty-dollar
expenditure questioned when you are looking at large holdings in investments and thousands in expenditures? The
court clerk assigned to review our yearly accounting decided
that a girl who was disabled didn't need a luxury purchase
from a jewelry store, and we were off on yet another costly
and time-consuming legal battle.

What was this *red flag* purchase? A quality constructed
medical ID bracelet that would withstand Jenn's rough use.
For the court to question a forty-dollar expenditure and
then spend thousands of dollars out of the trust for this
simple matter to be dragged through the court was ridiculous and unwarranted. I was furious, my pulse increased
a thousandfold as I read the letter requesting yet another
appearance before the court.

As Mark and I, our attorney, and the bank official filed
into the courtroom that day, it was hard to keep a calm
composure as I all too vividly remembered this routine.

I'd been warned that my appointment as a trustee was constantly being scrutinized to make sure funds were not being diverted for purposes other than for the beneficiary. I couldn't fathom how difficult it would be to run Jenn's programs and continue with the progress we were making if my control were challenged or taken away. It was terrifying and horrifying, and every nerve ending was on edge as I sat next to our lawyer and waited for the gavel to fall and potentially crush all my plans and efforts for Jenn.

Once the judge was seated, the court's attorney asked to make an opening statement.

"Your honor, I have carefully reviewed the annual accounting for this trust and find nothing remiss. I spoke with the defense's attorney and the jewelry purchase that was questioned was both appropriate and necessary. That purchase was in fact for a medical ID bracelet, something of great importance for the client to wear for her safety."

He continued on, "I feel there was an overreaction on the part of the court, a simple phone call by the county clerk to the bank trustees would have easily cleared this matter up, sparing the time and expense of a court appearance. I would suggest steps be taken in the future to prevent such a grossly misguided response to so small an expense or question."

Wow! I couldn't believe what my ears were hearing. This attorney had just reprimanded the court for poorly handling the case. Our attorney didn't have to say a word, the judge quickly ruled in our favor. But the bank and I did take away a clear message from both of our court appearances—we were being watched, and for our protection, we would need to take care to document everything.

THE BANK OFFICIALS were concerned about the watchful and suspicious eyes of the court on Jenn's finances. More than once, they reviewed with me their concern about using trust money for Jenn to purchase gifts for her family.

"We worry how the court will view these purchases," they commented.

I answered, "I understand, but Jenn should be allowed to have a normal life as long as she can afford it. In our culture, people buy gifts for each other for holidays and special occasions. Jenn's gifting is not extravagant and certainly doesn't put the trust's assets at risk of being depleted. The many steps that go into gifting all benefit her: the shopping, wrapping the package, and ultimately a wonderful happy interaction between her and the recipient when she gets to hand a gift to them. That should be all the justification needed for her to take part in this very normal activity. Are people who are disabled not allowed to participate in this kind of social interaction if they have enough funds to do so?"

"We see your point and think we can defend our position if questioned by the court," they said.

That was the response I'd hoped for.

In all fairness to the court, Jenn's was the first supplemental needs trust established in New York State and there was a steep learning curve for all concerned. It was important for us as trustees to help define and establish the guidelines of how these resources could and should be used to benefit the person they covered. We understood the need for the court to be concerned about abuses, especially if the funds were being depleted. But they also needed to understand that if funds were not being jeopardized, they had to give enough latitude to the trustees to ensure that a person who was disabled was not held in check from doing anything and everything other people might do. Fortunately, the gifting issue was never raised by the court. Perhaps they were a little more cautious after the scolding they received from their attorney about questioning small expenditures from the trust.

IT WASN'T JUST the court system we were battling. The New York State Department of Health had their eyes on Jenn's case as well. They pegged her as their number one person to repatriate back to New York State because of a new facility they'd opened in Duchess County. If she was moved, the Medicaid dollars spent in Connecticut would return back into the New York economy.

A New York State caseworker came to Danbury to review the status of Jenn's care and evaluate how they would replicate everything for her back in her home state. After years of developing the perfect placement for Jenn, all was in jeopardy because of a new facility that needed to fill beds.

The caseworker's review could not have been more glowing for the care Jenn was receiving, and her recommendation was for Jenn to remain in her current placement. In fact, her report included the remark, "New York will not be able to replicate the programs, living standards, and care that this client is receiving in her current placement."

The New York caseworker recognized the uniqueness and beauty of the life Jenn was living at Ability. But the state, steered more by budgets than by a person's welfare, continued their relentless pursuit of getting clients back into their territory, and in spite of the report, Jenn remained at the top of their list as a person to repatriate to New York. I wasn't having that!

It was time to call upon our representative in the state capital to help us deal with what would be a devastating move for Jenn. Mark and I set up an interview with our senator at his local office. He listened to our plight, really listened, nodding and shaking his head in disgust when we told him how New York wanted to move Jenn back in-state.

"Let me take care of it. As long as I am in office, she will stay right where she is," he promised us.

I don't know exactly who he spoke with or how he did it, but the results were profound. Suddenly the gears within the state government began moving to review the case, and New York State ultimately ruled that Jenn would remain in her current placement without the threat of repatriation. That was a monumental change, an unimaginable relief that I could hardly believe. As though by magic, the never-ending threat to Jennifer's placement that I worried about was whisked away, evaporating into thin air, and leaving me weightless in an atmosphere of no negative energy to pull me down.

JENN HAD BEEN my full-time job from day one of the accident. There was always a new battle to fight, more medical issues to address, a staff position to fill, and meetings and conferences to attend. I spent hours on the computer preparing spreadsheets and researching the professionals I needed to consult. Determined to give our daughter the best benefits and opportunities available required the drive of an unrelenting mother, and a supportive father who was still working to provide for us. The battles were wearing on a family who had experienced so much, but each challenge gave us insight about possible creative solutions if we drew upon our considerable determination and resilience. Each battle won and every positive outcome attained encouraged us to never give up on anything that would make life better for Jennifer. Rather than breaking us down, the battles we fought empowered us.

Chapter 14

THE BOISVERTS

I was impressed with Christine Boisvert from the first time I met her ten years ago when we brought Jenn to Squire. Chris was twenty-one years old, and right away we recognized her vibrance and energy along with her kindness and empathy toward our family and the other clients at the group home. Once she became part of Jenn's personal staff, it was fun to discover the depth of her character beyond what we had seen on those first days and weeks as we were getting to know her. Humor, a strong and enduring sense of direction, trustworthiness, and dedication to people with disabilities were among her many trademarks.

The first year Chris started working with Jenn, we were invited to Louisiana to attend a big family Christmas celebration hosted by my cousins. We didn't imagine that we could possibly go to this function, as we always had Jenn home with us during holidays. When Chris heard about our awkward situation, she volunteered to take Jenn home over the holiday and allow us the freedom to attend our family event.

We appreciated her offer, but initially hesitated because this would be the first time Jenn stayed overnight at a staff member's house. Although the daily routines would be similar, we were not sure about the nights. We all had a particular concern about whether Jenn would sleep through the night or get up to roam through the house and possibly become disoriented. The stairway next to the kitchen in Chris's bilevel home also presented a safety concern.

When Maria took Jenn on overnight trips, the hotel rooms had no kitchen or stairways to worry about. When Jenn stayed with us, Mark always slept on the floor in her bedroom, so he'd know if she got up. At Squire an overnight shift of staff was awake at all times and could look out for Jenn, but this would not be the case at Chris's house. None of us took lightly the risks of the new plan.

Chris offered assurances that all was going to be okay. "Maria is going to stay over too, so she'll be an extra set of eyes and helping hands with Jenn. She'll sleep with Jenn on the pullout sofa in the living room and will know if Jenn gets up during the night. She's taken her on many overnight trips and looks forward to spending the holiday with my family." All this was spoken with an air of confidence that gave me little to worry about as Mark, Amy, and I headed to Louisiana.

After we returned, I was anxious to see Jenn and hear about her overnight adventure. I had checked in by phone while we were gone and had good reports, but I still needed the face-to-face confirmation that all was well.

Chris was excited to fill me in on the whole story of Christmas at the Boisverts. "Everything went perfectly, and Jenn slept through the night. Maria was very helpful with dinner preparations, and my family loved having Jenn and her join in our celebration. It made the holiday all the more special. When I first suggested the idea of Jenn staying over, I was more nervous than I let on to you, Barb. Maria kept telling me not to worry and that it would be fine, but I didn't want anything to get screwed up. As Maria predicted, everything went smoothly, and I look forward to the next time Jenn stays at my house."

Although it was unusual for us not to have Jenn with us over Christmas, our absence paved the way for many wonderful experiences Jenn would have going forward at other peoples' homes. It was the start of a new and meaningful routine in her care—weekends and sleepovers with the Boisverts and Benzes.

AS THE YEARS passed, I came to think of Chris as the girl who never grew up. For as long as I'd known her, she'd expressed a love for all things related to holidays, from dressing up for Halloween and artfully carving pumpkins, to making creative eggs for Easter. Chris never outgrew amusement park rides and adored Disney World. She'd come back from a visit to The Magic Kingdom with her family and be all aglow telling me about the perfect vacation they'd had. Given the option, I think Chris would have been perfectly happy to live in Cinderella's Castle with Goofy and Mickey as her neighbors and friends. This charming aspect of her personality lent itself well to make her a fun companion for Jenn and helped Mark and me feel confident that she would bring a lighter, brighter side to Jenn's daily routines.

Chris celebrated all the holidays and special events with the enthusiasm of an adult who loved the playful side of life. She took the liberty to make the kid in all of us come to the surface and join in the fun.

The week before Halloween in 2003, ten years after Jenn arrived at Squire, I visited just in time to see staff and clients decorate the group home for the holiday. Fake spider webs were carefully draped over the front shrubbery and cornstalks were tied to the front porch posts. Colorful gourds and an array of pumpkins were arranged around the lamppost next to the driveway. Inside the house, monster plastic spiders graced the corners of the living room walls while paper black cats and witches peered across the room from the bookshelves and coffee table. I could feel the excitement in the air as Squire was transformed into a festive display of traditional holiday colors and fare. But no Halloween was complete without a few jack-o-lanterns to reside next to the cornstalks outside, and Chris made sure that element was also tended to.

"I love pumpkin carving," Chris said as she arranged all the items needed to help Jenn artfully carve the jack-o-lanterns. "Jenn doesn't necessarily share that fascination, but I expect her to help anyway. Her job is to remove all the slimy seed gunk once I cut open the top."

I loved watching Jenn and Chris work on this project at the kitchen table at Squire. I manned the camera as Jenn dug into the soft pumpkin shell to clean out the innards. This was a challenge for her as she wasn't one for getting her hands dirty, or having wet, slimy things touch her fingers. But when she wore disposable gloves, she was ready to dive in and do what was needed to get the job done.

As she removed each handful of muck, she energetically shook the seeds off her gloves before reaching back into the pumpkin for more. "Jenn, wipe them off on the paper towel, that's what it's for," Chris directed. Jenn gave Chris a smile, wiped a few seeds on the paper towels but then reverted back to flinging the rest of them in all directions around the room. Carving pumpkins can be messy in any circumstance, but this went far beyond the norm—seeds were on the counters, the floors, and us. The one place you didn't find any seeds was on those gloves.

As they worked on their project, Jenn's happiness was written all over her face. Her giggles and the big belly laughs that repeatedly burst out of her further confirmed the fun she was having. But as I watched, my mind slipped back to the magical time long ago when I did this same activity with my young girls. I missed those days; I longed for them, but I couldn't let my face reveal where my thoughts had taken me.

Each year Ability, the corporate facility that Squire was part of, sponsored a costume dance party at their main building for all clients and staff. Chris and her cohort, Joe, made sure everyone from Squire was properly outfitted with skillfully crafted Halloween garb.

Two days after the party I went to visit Jenn. Upon entering the door at Squire, Chris was quick to point out the framed collage of pictures taken at the event. As I looked at the photos, I marveled at their creativity in making all those perky outfits; everyone looked ghoulishly delightful. But slowly another familiar moment of despair seeped into my psyche as I took in the reality of what those photos represented. This was not the group I had once imagined Jenn to be a part of at this point in her life. She should have been posing in the pictures with her own family, a husband and children, not with people who lived and worked in a group home with her. I found some satisfaction in her smile, but I experienced an underlying current of sadness that discolored the happiness exhibited in the matted photos displayed for all to see.

It had been twelve years since Jenn's accident, but I still

harbored a feeling of loss and turmoil for the daughter who should have been, while faced with the one staring back at me from the photos. I worked at being upbeat around others. I didn't want them to see my emotional despair, so I planted a smile on my face and moved forward, burying the darkness deep inside. I would share these hidden sorrows with my husband once I returned home. Like me, he realized with each passing year that the life Jenn should have had was not the one she was living.

"Where did you guys get all these costumes?" I questioned as I studied each outfit I saw in the photos. There was an impressive Count Dracula, a couple of zombies, and a few more endearing characters like Elvis, Minnie Mouse, and The Cat in the Hat. Jenn was outfitted as Dorothy from the Wizard of Oz. I'd made costumes for my girls when they were little, but they were nothing compared to these amazing works of art.

"We mostly picked stuff up at Goodwill, but some things we got from the Halloween store," Joe replied.

They found gowns and suits that, in the spirit of Michael Jackson's "Thriller" music video, were adapted for the zombies and ghouls in the lineup. Their tattered attire and face paint made them look like they had just risen from the dead. The group's Dracula had fake blood dripping down his white shirt and standing next to him was a bride with a blood-stained gown who was apparently part of the carnage.

Chris wore her favorite disguise as the Wicked Witch of the West, dressed completely in black, with green face paint, a black wig, and a massive black witch's hat. Of course, Jenn served as Chris's counterpart— Dorothy. With her hair braided and hanging down over each shoulder, wearing a blue-and-white-gingham dress from the Halloween store, and carrying a basket containing a stuffed dog, Jenn looked perfect in her role as the girl from Kansas.

CHRIS WORKED MANY different shifts and often stepped in to cover for others. The overtime pay was a nice incentive, but she always told me she didn't mind having Jenn for the extra time either. "Because I can bring her home, the added hours don't take time away from my kids," she often reminded me.

When Chris's sons, Ian and Aaron—identical twins—were toddlers, their mom and Jenn picked them up at the daycare center and brought them back to Squire to hang out while their mom finished her shift.

Fortunately for the boys, there was an ample supply of toys in Jenn's room. They were actually her learning materials but were age appropriate for the entertainment of the twins too: Legos, puzzles, crayons, scissors, markers, and building blocks, just to name a few. With free access to all the neat stuff in Jenn's closet, they never complained about being at Squire. Chris would tell me how they loved raiding Aunt Jenn's closet full of stuff and also enjoyed interacting with the other staff and clients in the group home. They were often there when I was visiting and, like their mom, were fun to talk to. It was deeply touching to see how they always made sure to acknowledge each client who was hanging out in the kitchen or living room before disappearing into Jenn's room down the hallway.

When Ian and Aaron were in kindergarten, Chris had to pick them up at the school bus stop each afternoon. This was during Chris's shift, so Aunt Jenn was always with her, and the foursome would be together for the remainder of the day whether it was running errands, shopping, or hanging out at home until they brought Jenn back to Squire Court in the early evening.

"It's so cute how excited the boys are to see Jenn, and for her to see them, when we go to pick them up from the bus stop," Chris told me. "They run to the car, first giving me a hug, and then they turn to Jenn and hug her too. She gives them each a pat on the head and grabs their lunch box to see if they have any goodies left inside. She must smell the food or something, but the only thing she ever finds are empty wrappers. After she checks out one lunch box, she's ready to check out the other. The boys think she's funny; they start cracking up, and Jenn joins in with the laughs."

By the time their sister, Lily, arrived in the family seven years later, the boys were older and less interested in the toys in Jenn's room. They'd spend their time at Squire doing homework and goofing around with staff and clients.

As Lily grew into a delightful little girl, she was not particularly interested in Jenn's room as her brothers had been. Instead, when at Squire, she'd talk with everyone and often give a performance of her latest dance moves or sing her favorite song for them using a pretend microphone.

Like her brothers, little sister Lily loved Aunt Jenn. Chris was always bringing me stories about the two of them. One that stands out was when Jenn and Chris went to pick Lily up from preschool. In her eagerness to get to Jenn and give her a big hug, Lily caught her off balance and accidentally knocked her down. Lily cried, devastated that she may have hurt Aunt Jenn. She was all over her beloved family member showering her with hugs and kisses and frantically repeating, "I'm sorry!"

Chris said that Jenn seemed a little shell-shocked that this tiny three-year-old was able to bring her down to the pavement, but all seemed to be forgiven after the initial yell of disbelief and irritation from the surprised Aunt Jenn. Lily tried to help her mom get Jenn up. With a leg brace and compromised right arm, Jenn was like dead weight to lift off the ground, although she was able to get herself up if she wanted to.

"She was not going to help at all," Chris told me. "Lily was trying to help, but basically I had to lift Jenn up off the ground by myself. As I lifted her, she started laughing. I told her, 'Okay, Jenn, now you are being a brat.' But I was glad she found the situation funny."

One of my favorite stories about Lily and Jenn was Lily asking Chris why Aunt Jenn had more bellybuttons than her. As a fellow female, Lily was there while mom gave Jenn a bath in the morning after a sleepover. Sure enough, directly above Jenn's bellybutton was another hole in her abdomen, the place where the feeding tube was inserted after her accident. It did indeed look like another bellybutton! This was a complicated question for Chris to answer, but she came up with a response that made perfect sense to her little girl. "Lily, Aunt Jenn is special, that is why she is lucky enough to have an extra bellybutton."

In Lily's eyes, Aunt Jenn *was* special, so there you have it; special people have extra bellybuttons. Chris could see that, for Lily, Aunt Jenn was fun to have around as another girl to balance the effect of having two brothers in the house. She expected Jenn to play with her and always brought toys over to engage her in a game or activity. Sometimes Jenn was more compliant than others, and often she didn't understand what was expected of her. That would confuse Lily—she didn't comprehend that, because of a disability, Jenn sometimes didn't know how to play correctly. This was humorously evident when Chris showed me a video she took of the two girls playing with Lily's new Barbie doll house.

In the video, Chris helped Jenn to sit down on the floor as Lily excitedly started setting up for a pretend party at Barbie's house. Jenn was smiling and giggling, more than willing to participate in this activity, but she seemed to have devised a plan of her own— stack all the furniture in one of the playhouse rooms. She quickly gathered every piece of furniture that Lily had carefully placed around the playhouse and added them to her rapidly overflowing room, one piece on top of the other. This was not what three-year-old Lily had in mind, and it quickly led to her total meltdown.

"She isn't playing right," Lily screamed as she stormed out of view of the camera. With Lily gone, Jenn finished stacking the furniture, put all the miniature dolls in another room, and closed up the playhouse—all was cleaned up nice and neat. Chris on the other end of the camera could be heard laughing and trying to explain to Lily what just happened.

"Lil, come back, Aunt Jenn thought she was helping. Can you teach her how to play with the Barbies the right way? She doesn't know how."

With that, the camera footage ended. Chris assured me that as always, Lily was quick to forgive and soon came back for more playtime, as usual with a better attitude. It seemed that, for Jenn's part, nothing strange had happened. She appeared to have had a good time and was more than ready to try the next activity that Lily might offer.

There were some things that Aunt Jenn wasn't thrilled about but at times would tolerate. Lily liked to practice braiding hair, and Jenn was okay with a few minutes of this girly activity. When Chris detected that Jenn was no longer happy with the pretend beauty shop routine, she would try to get them to switch it up and have Jenn braid Lily's hair. "Barb, it is so cute to see the two of them interact," she told me. "One is no better at braiding than the other, but I assured both of them that they were doing a top-notch job."

AS THE KIDS grew older and became more involved in after-school activities, it was hard for the family to always have a sit-down dinner. Ian was into sports, and Aaron was involved in the local art studio. But Wednesdays were different: that was always the day Mom brought Jenn home, and the whole family was together to share a meal, sometimes for the first time that week.

Because of Chris's ability to bring her work home, there was added stability in the Boisvert family. Getting to activities, school pickups, snow days, or conference days never presented a problem for her. Chris could serve as mom and caregiver at the same time.

Chris told me, "This blend of work and family has big benefits beyond what I first imagined. Convenience and a larger paycheck are obvious perks, but the compassionate lessons of tolerance and acceptance my kids learned from Jenn was something I had not anticipated. It all came together very naturally and unknowingly. Ian, Aaron, and Lily have come to love your daughter and accept her as part of our family."

Jenn reaped a huge benefit from this scenario too—regular involvement with a loving family who deeply cared for and understood her.

ON ONE OF my visits to see Jenn, Chris brought in pictures of a new addition to her family. She had mentioned various times that she was looking for a family pet and was excited to show me the picture of Jenn holding her new puppy.

"The kids and I named her Daisy," Chris said like a proud new parent. She had been searching the internet for weeks and was thrilled when she found what was sure to be the perfect pet for her family—a golden labradoodle. This hypoallergenic breed was ideal because it wouldn't trigger the boys' allergies.

"I took Jenn with me to pick Daisy up from the breeder. Not even the kids knew I was going to get her. On the ride home, I put the puppy in the backseat with Jenn. Even though Daisy was in a carrier, Jenn kept up her moaning groans of protest each time the puppy became too excited or started whining or barking."

"Jenn, she's scared, just pet her," Chris said from the driver's seat. "But Jenn kept up her grumbly noises and moved herself as far away from the carrier as her seatbelt would allow.

"When we got back to my house, we left the puppy in her crate while we went to pick up the kids from the school bus stop. As we walked in the front door, the first thing they saw was a puppy sitting in a crate next to the coffee table in the living room. They were so excited to get their hands on her and could hardly wait their turn while one of the others was holding her. All of us were busy oohing and aahing as we watched each move Daisy made while we played and cuddled with her. Of course, Jenn was way more interested in a snack which was part of the after-school routine. She was hanging out in the kitchen, and I am sure wondering what all the fuss was about. She was definitely not interested in hovering over some silly dog."

As the months passed, Daisy outgrew the puppy stage, and Jenn slowly became more tolerant of her. In fact, whenever Jenn stayed over at the Boisverts' house, she shared the living room sofa bed with Daisy, who always slept with Chris unless Jenn was staying over. For some unknown reason, Daisy was drawn to Jenn like a magnet. If Jenn was sitting on the sofa, Daisy would jump up and lay down beside her. Jenn would gently pet her, and over time, the two became good buddies.

A favorite story in the Boisvert family, told to me numerous times, was the day Aaron made a birthday cake for Daisy. This yummy treat was filled with peanut butter and carrots, suitable for a dog and family alike. Everyone was looking forward to making a big deal over Daisy's first birthday and presenting her with a piece of the specially prepared cake. Star-shaped and complete with a candle, it was the result of Aaron's artistic and culinary talents. Just before it was to be served, the family was distracted by something and left the kitchen momentarily unguarded. That was just the opportunity Jenn was waiting for. In a matter of seconds, she consumed two entire legs of the scrumptious star-shaped cake. Fortunately, Daisy wasn't any the wiser about her notably smaller dessert, and the episode gave the rest of the family something to laugh about. The Boisverts still chuckle when they recall the guilty look on Jenn's face as she tried to pretend that nothing had happened.

EVERY TIME I listened to Chris's stories of Jenn and her time with the Boisvert family, it never failed to make my day. The love and kindness shown to my daughter when she was with them was beyond measure. It exceeded my hopes and dreams for her, and I was thrilled at the wonder of it all. This was Jenn's new life.

Chapter 15

THE BENZ FAMILY

When I reflected back over the ten years that Suzanne Benz was part of our team as one of Jenn's personal caregivers, I could see Jenn had grown as close to Suzanne and her family as she had with Christine's. With time, I learned how Jenn interacted with the Benzes through the interesting stories they regularly shared with me on my visits to Squire. I enjoyed these tales, as they brought me into Jenn's life when I was away from her and allowed me to better see into the world she was immersed in with her caretakers.

As I got to know Suzanne, I found her to be an open book and more than willing to fill me in on her past and especially how the relationship with her husband, Scott, evolved.

"I've lived in Danbury, Connecticut, my whole life and have no plans to live anywhere else. I need to live in the same town as my parents. It seems like the right thing to do, and I wouldn't have it any other way," she laughingly told me. Luckily, this was the same place she met the love of her life, Scott, who had also grown up in Danbury and had his roots firmly planted in Connecticut soil.

Scott was a big guy with a cherubic face, shaved head, and more than a few tattoos hidden under the Honda uniform he wore so proudly. Suzanne shared with me a little history of her beloved husband. "In his younger days, he was a real troublemaker. In school he was every teacher's worst nightmare, and as a young adult, he was a guy who loved to go drinking with his buddies—an honest man who was living life on the edge." But all that changed when he started dating Suzanne, a single mom who altered the course of his life.

Suzanne, in contrast, was a responsible, hardworking parent, and mature beyond her years. But Scott made her laugh and showed promise in his dedication to both her and her young daughter, Mary. "He had to change his lifestyle and grow up before I'd let him become part of my life," Suzanne said. "He was a fun-loving, big-hearted guy whose unruly high school reputation was well-known, even to me."

In Suzanne, Scott must have seen all the possibilities life offered if he wanted family, love, and stability. Few who knew him in his younger years would have placed him in a happy marriage, credited him with being a great father, or foreseen him in a responsible position of management at Honda of Danbury.

FROM SUZANNE, I learned about Jenn's special connection with Scott. "When Jenn is at my house for the afternoon and evening, she seems aware of when it is about time for Scott to come walking in the front door after a long day at work. She has a particular corner wall next to the kitchen that she leans on during her wait for him. From there she can watch me preparing the meal and still keep an eye on the front door for the arrival of the man of the house.

"There is a nervous energy in Jenn as she hangs out by the wall, probably because she is thinking about eating. She picked at the corner of the wall until she chipped off a bit of paint. Barb, I tried to get her to stop, but the next time she waited for Scott, she was back at it. As the habit continued, the chipped area grew larger. We decided as a family to just look at it as a fond etching left by our dear friend—couldn't stop it so figured we might as well embrace it.

"Jenn always has a larger-than-life greeting saved for Scott when he finally walks through the front door. In a flash, she rushes over, grabs his hand, and directs him to the kitchen table."

Scott told me more than once with a chuckle, "I love her enthusiasm for dinner; Jenn and I think alike."

It wasn't long after Suzanne started working with Jenn that she began bringing her home for overnight stays. She loved to fill me in on how things went the next time I saw her after one of these overnights. Suzanne was a storyteller, so sharing details of what happened at home with Jenn was right up her alley.

In Scott and Suzanne's first house, the bedrooms were located on the second level. "In the beginning, I slept with Jenn on the foldout couch on the first floor, but eventually I became comfortable with the situation and let Jenn spend the night alone on the sleeper sofa. With a motion detector set up at the doorway to the kitchen, I felt we had all bases covered to keep her safe. It only took a couple of times of the alarm going off and her being caught in the kitchen for Jenn to give up on the idea of nocturnal food cruising and let everyone sleep peacefully through the night. Unfortunately for Scott, that meant he couldn't sneak into the kitchen for a late snack either."

In their second home, Jenn slept in the basement—Scott's man-cave—on that same pullout sofa as in the first house. "There is really nothing troublesome for Jenn to get into down there. With the kitchen one level above her, we have the motion detector set at the top of the stairway so it will go off if she crosses the threshold to the upstairs."

Scott found the new arrangement to be a winning proposition. Although displaced from his man-cave, he was equipped with a TV on the first floor and had easy access to his kitchen without tripping the alarm. In a short time, Jenn realized that she would not be able to sneak into the kitchen while at the Benzes, so she settled into her basement bedroom and would not appear until everyone was up the next morning.

SCOTT FELT HE and Jenn communicated on a deep level. "There were no unanswered questions between Jenn and me," he told me. "I knew what she was thinking. There was no need for words. We both understood all there was to know about each other."

To Scott, Jenn's messages were always clear and precise. "I knew what Jenn wanted when she greeted me at the door—we were both hungry and ready to eat. There wasn't any need to guess Jenn's thoughts when she wanted more food and someone said, 'No!' It was pretty clear that she wasn't happy about that. If she stood by the front door with a persuading look on her face and a nod of the head, you knew she was ready to leave. In the cold months, Jenn might put on her gloves even indoors which meant that she was obviously cold. How much more clearly could she have expressed herself?"

All of Scott's close friends knew Jenn quite well; she was always there whether they were coming by for a videogame night, Super Bowl Sunday, a party, or for a random drop-in visit. In fact, she was so much a part of the Benz family that Jenn was often invited to parties hosted by Scott's friends or even their kids. This girl who was disabled was so tightly woven into Scott's life that even his friends could not separate her from their own family gatherings.

The bond between the Benzes and Jenn's own family— us—took time and shared events to develop. The stories Suzanne shared with me over our weekly lunches when I came to visit Jenn painted a colorful picture of Scott and the inner workings of the Benz family. Suzanne would relay stories about our family to Scott: what we were like and what was going on in our lives. In this way, through Suzanne, all of us felt like we knew a lot about each other, even though we didn't have many opportunities to be together in the early years.

SUZANNE'S DAUGHTER, MARY, was five years old when her mom started working with Jenn in 1998. She had long, flowing, dark hair and beautiful brown eyes. She was a slender, wispy child who was always friendly but a bit reserved until her teen years.

When she was about sixteen, Mary told me, "My memory doesn't go back to a time when Aunt Jenn wasn't in my life. She was always a member of my family. Her unique laugh was always heard in my house during all of my growing up years."

She went on to say, "If my friends were going to meet her for the first time, I'd keep it simple as far as Jenn was concerned. I'd just tell them that Jenn was part of the family—she doesn't talk, and she makes noises. My friends accepted that this was how Jenn was, and we'd continue on with whatever we planned to do."

Mary told me how the routines went. "When it was dinner time, Jenn had a place at our table where she always sat. Just like the rest of us, she was expected to be at the table, and when she wasn't, we missed her. Having Jenn with us never seemed like work; she was just someone we all helped take care of just as we would any other member of our family because we loved her," Mary told me.

"You could tell that Jenn understood everything going on around her as she expressed her emotions very clearly. You knew when she was sad, mad, happy, and excited."

Mary continued, "Holidays were the best if Jenn was there. She added lots of extra laughs and unexpected hilarity with all her silly antics. We always waited until she could be with us to trim the Christmas tree, carve our Halloween pumpkins, or color Easter eggs. Having her with us at those times made everything feel complete and right."

As she was growing up, Mary viewed herself as a happy child, always smiling and laughing. "Life was good. I had everything any kid needed to be content. But I did question why God would let such a bad thing happen to Jenn. It was hard for me as a young kid to understand such a thing."

Mary wasn't alone in trying to understand why Jenn had been so severely injured. I struggled with the same question myself, especially right after Jenn's accident when she was in a coma. A family friend, who was also a clergyman, often came to the hospital to visit Mark and me and confessed even his lack of understanding on such matters. On one of his visits, he brought a book for Mark and me to read: *Why Do Bad Things Happen to Good People* by David Arnold. This book proved to be a source of great comfort to me. The author made me see that both good and bad exist in our world, but we would not recognize one without the other because both of them are necessary for us to appreciate the difference. I came to the conclusion that the accident wasn't God's doing but a result of human actions. It was possible He intervened when Jenn's life was in the balance between life and death, but that was beyond anything I could state as provable fact. Mary's question was a valid one. I shared some of the ideas with her that I took from the book and hoped they would in time help her come to terms with her very profound question.

DIANNA, SUZANNE'S MIDDLE child, had golden blonde hair and fair skin like her father. With her bubbly personality, she was more animated than her siblings and brought a lot of energy into any gathering. Dianna was closest in age to Chris's daughter, Lily. These two girls connected right away when the families were brought together. Lily enjoyed having someone to hang out with who was like an older sister to her, and Dianna was always eager to do things with Lily, as they had many of the same interests, especially dancing. Whenever I saw them together, they were always showing each other the latest dance moves they were working on along with a few gymnastic flips and handstands.

Unlike Chris and Suzanne's other kids who saw Jenn as a playmate, Dianna at an early age liked to take on a mothering role. I saw this when we were at the beach house each summer.

I remember the time Dianna decided it was time to put on Jenn's shoes.

"Here, Aunt Jenn, I'll help you," spoke the reassuring voice of five-year-old Dianna.

It was a struggle for us adults to get Jenn's braced foot into her shoe and Dianna didn't have the strength needed to successfully maneuver the inflexible device and foot into the shoe opening, but she made up for it in sheer resolve. Jenn was cooperating as best she could as little Dianna struggled with the big shoes in her small hands, but patience was not one of Jenn's virtues, and her smile quickly turned into a grimace as she started groaning about all the pushing and shoving going on with her feet. Undeterred, Dianna persisted until Jenn grabbed a shoe and threw it across the room.

"Dianna, why don't you let me do Aunt Jenn's shoes?" Suzanne suggested.

"But I want to help dress Aunt Jenn."

"How about if I put her shoes on, and you tie the laces?" Suzanne offered. Dianna seemed pleased with the compromise, and once Suzanne finished her part of the task, Dianna slowly managed to get the laces in a reasonable semblance of a bow.

"Can I do her hair?" asked her determined young daughter. "I can put it in a ponytail."

"If Aunt Jenn will sit still for you to do it, why not?" Suzanne said with a shrug of her shoulders.

No sooner were the words out of Suzanne's mouth than Dianna, with hairbrush in hand, started gently smoothing out Jenn's tangled locks. I have to admit, I didn't think Dianna was going to be any more successful with doing Jenn's hair than with her shoes, but I was wrong. Ever so carefully, Dianna managed to get at least most of the knots out of Jenn's hair and had the hair bunched up in a ponytail. Was it perfect? No. Off center and drooping a bit because the hair-tie wasn't tight enough, but I still had to give the young beautician credit for completing the task she'd set out to do.

In the years to come, Dianna would become very accomplished at styling hair, especially when it came to braiding. Jenn often had a beautiful French braid when she stayed with the Benzes or when we were at the beach house thanks to Dianna. But it wasn't just Jenn's hair that had Dianna's attention. She was always looking for ways to help care for Aunt Jenn and was glad to step in to assist without even being asked: lending a hand getting Jenn up and down stairs, redirecting her away from the stove, or wrapping her in a beach towel to keep the sun's rays off her legs. Dianna's devotion to my daughter was evident and unwavering. I marveled at the beauty of watching Dianna lovingly oversee her Aunt Jenn's care and well-being and seeing how this interaction was so positively molding her compassion for those who are disabled.

JACKSON, WITH HIS dark hair and sturdy build, looked a lot like his mom, Suzanne, and her Italian side of the family. He was the youngest sibling of the Benz family and the most even-tempered child I ever knew. Did this have something to do with having two older sisters?

Jackson told me that as a little kid, he didn't realize there was anything wrong with Aunt Jenn. "I remember going into her room at Squire and thought we were having a normal conversation as she showed me some of her stuff. It wasn't until I was older that I realized she was different from other adults."

A favorite story about Jackson and Jenn came about when he was still a little guy and the proud owner of a child-sized motorized Hummer truck that he loved to drive around in the front yard. Knowing Jenn found this to be particularly funny as she watched him maneuver his vehicle from place to place, Suzanne and Scott thought she should join him as a passenger. With video camera in hand, Suzanne began rolling the tape as Scott brought Jenn over to the Hummer and encouraged her to hop in with his son. I loved watching the video when Suzanne brought it to Squire for me to see.

"Get in Jenn, Jackson will take you for a ride," Scott said as he gave her a helping hand and she wedged herself in the seat next to her small driver. Laughing the whole time, it seemed as though she had been waiting all along for the opportunity to do this. There was no hesitation on her part.

Jackson had a big smile planted on his face and was happy to give Aunt Jenn a ride in his dream vehicle. Scott backed away and slowly Jackson started driving across the front yard. Jenn gave a big wave to Suzanne and the camera and seemed to be acknowledging that all was good, and this was as much fun as she anticipated.

Both Scott and Suzanne saw what was coming next before it happened—the small ledge that separated the driveway from the yard loomed in the path of the approaching Hummer. "Turn Jackson, turn the wheel," Scott and Suzanne yelled. Too late! In slow motion, the Hummer banged down on the driveway with a sharp thud. Jenn let out a loud unhappy yell as she gave Jackson an alarmed and disgusted look. Afterward, he didn't seem to understand the harm in what he'd done. Apparently he'd driven over the ledge more than once and saw nothing wrong with it.

"Jackson, you can't drive over the ledge with Jenn; you scared her," Scott explained to his son, who'd just shrugged his shoulders. But Jenn was done. Looking disgusted, she started to get out, and Scott was quickly at her side to help her step out of the vehicle. "It's okay, Jenn, you can ride some more," he tried to explain. But Jenn ignored Scott's plea and quickly started walking toward the house. Clearly, she wasn't getting back in with this reckless stunt driver.

Along with showing me the video, Suzanne gave me an adorable picture that she'd taken of their escapade: Jenn towering over Jackson in the mini vehicle. They truly looked like they were sitting in a clown car, Jenn with her arm around Jackson pulling him in close to her and both with big smiles on their faces.

JENN ALWAYS SPENT the Fourth of July with the Benzes, along with Christine's family, and on occasion we joined them too. There was always a large gathering for this yearly holiday celebration at Suzanne's parents' home. Friends and family were invited to this extravaganza whose guest list numbered over a hundred attendees. For days, Suzanne and her mom prepared the food, as this was not a catered affair; everything was homemade and in great abundance. Jenn played a part in the food preparation too. Her specialty was the cracking and peeling of hard-boiled eggs for Suzanne to make into deviled eggs. Jenn loved this task and was a most willing participant.

The day of the event, party tents were set up in the backyard for shade or if needed in the event of rain. Scott was assigned to the grill with hot dogs, hamburgers, and filet mignon demanding his attention from early afternoon until late in the evening. Family and friends arrived bringing side dishes of pasta, salad, and baked beans as well as desserts of every kind. This was truly a feast. Tray after tray of hot meats and dishes were set atop Sterno burners and lined up over several long tables on the backyard deck. Side dishes were arranged in front of those trays, leaving little open space on the tables as all the food was made ready for eager guests.

Although most guests would be found outside in the sunshine, Jenn liked to hang out with Suzanne's Aunt Maria at the kitchen table. People always wanted to feed Jenn because she would get so excited about it, but with her dietary restrictions in place, everyone followed the rules, except for Aunt Maria. She just couldn't resist the temptation to get the smiles and giggles of joy from Jenn each time she gave her a tasty morsel. "Oh, come on Suzanne, she can have this one little bite."

"No," Suzanne would affirm, "she has to wait for dinner." But as soon as Suzanne turned her back, Aunt Maria would slip Jenn something else to eat. Suzanne decided the best solution was to put healthy foods in proximity to Aunt Maria and Jenn because these two were in cahoots and thoroughly enjoying themselves. Jenn had Aunt Maria pegged as her favorite relative and would always stay at her side whenever there was a family gathering.

JENN'S LIFE WAS rich with people, love, and stimulating days filled with new adventures or just simple daily routines. She was free from worry about wars, climate change, politics, poverty, or epidemics. Hers was a life spent in the moment, untroubled by worldly matters. Her interests centered around food and the people she interacted with throughout the day. Mark and I recognized how fortunate she was to have the Benz and Boisvert families as part of her circle of support and love. They accepted and valued her as a fellow human being. These two families were giving Jenn the best life we could have hoped for.

Chapter 16

JENN IN
PUBLIC PLACES

The Ability clients regularly patronized local businesses for entertainment and shopping needs, but few of them had the one-on-one staff or private transportation to take advantage of these offerings the way Jenn did. She was a frequent visitor to the bowling alley, mall arcade, grocery stores, pharmacies, movie theaters, Michael's art supply, Staples, car wash, and of course, given how much she loved food, lots of restaurants.

One business that we frequented weekly was Bagelman, a cute eatery with great food in Brookfield, Connecticut's Candlewood Plaza. It was conveniently close to the group home, and the employees were always welcoming. On certain days of the week, Chris's and Suzanne's hours overlapped during lunch. I tried to be there on those days so I could spend time with both of them to hatch plans for the future and brainstorm, vent, chit-chat, and strategize while enjoying each other's company.

As Jenn happily munched on her sandwich and watched the busy people around her, I would catch up on things happening at the group home, in our private lives, and in the world at large.

We loved Bagelman and patronized them many times through the years. But not all businesses were accepting of Jenn and her loud noises, especially restaurants. Any place associated with food brought out the worst in her. There were times when Chris and Suzanne realized she was just too excitable to enter an eatery, so they would pass it by. At other times, everything seemed okay in the car, but her noises would escalate as they walked across the parking lot to the café, and they'd have to redirect her back to the car. Only if Jenn exhibited control and her vocalizations were at an acceptable volume would she be allowed to enter a restaurant.

Chris and Suzanne told me, "We dread the times when we are asked to leave a restaurant or are sent to a closed section to keep us isolated and far away from other patrons. We know the rejection isn't directed toward us—it's toward Jennifer. The idea that anyone would be intolerant of a person with special needs is just heartbreaking."

"What if Jenn understands what is being said to us?" they wondered out loud. "Does she know that others are judging her as different and therefore unacceptable?"

These worries brought tears to the eyes of both Chris and Suzanne. "How can people be so insensitive? Don't they understand that this person is just happy to be there and is excited to eat? Doesn't this special person have the right to come into an establishment and be served the same as anyone else?"

A situation that brought these concerns to light took place at a local restaurant, one often frequented by Suzanne's family. The owner made the mistake of seating Suzanne and Jenn in a separate room away from the other patrons. A few days later, she told me the whole story as tears came to her eyes.

"Jenn and I had gone there for dinner many times because the waitresses were always so nice, and we never had any problems. This time when we went in, instead of seating us in the dining room, the owner sat us by the front window where there were three or four booths. He sat us there, where nobody else was. There was plenty of space in the dining room, as there wasn't anything special going on at the time. Jenn was so good that day because she knew what to expect there. When she knew what was expected of her, she tended to be quieter. It's like that for anyone."

I listened, knowing the direction that this was going—an uncomfortable place, one of hurt and pain.

Her story continued, "I hadn't seen my kids that day because I left early and wasn't there when school let out. Scott called and said he and the kids were out, and they were going to swing by to say hi to us. When they came in, Dianna asked, 'Why are you guys sitting here when everyone else is sitting in the other room?' She wanted to know if I had asked to sit there, I told her no.

"It started to bother me that my daughter noticed something didn't seem right. If Jenn had been loud, I would have understood why they might stick us off to the side, but she was good when we walked into the restaurant. That Dianna noticed something was so obviously wrong really bothered me. Scott started to get annoyed about it too, and then I got mad, so upset that I couldn't eat. That never happens—I can always eat. Jenn, of course, ate. It didn't affect her at all, and she got a visit from Scott and the kids along with her meal.

"After a short time, Scott and the kids left, and Jenn finished eating, so it was time to pay the bill and go. The owner was the one at the cash register waiting to take our money. At this point, I was really mad. If even my kids, who know nothing, realized that for no apparent reason we were put to the side and not seated with everyone else, I had to confront him.

"'May I ask you why you seated us away from the other patrons, because your waitresses always seat us in the dining room? Your staff are always very nice, and we've always had an enjoyable time here.'

"'I have the right to seat you wherever I want,' he said bluntly.

"That rubbed me the wrong way. He could have said almost anything other than that, and he wasn't nice about it either. I told him he was rude and ignorant. Ignorant is a word I use when people don't understand how to be tolerant and appreciate someone with special needs. I repeated to him that he was extremely ignorant, and we'd never come back. He couldn't have cared less. When I left there, I didn't want to return to Squire yet because I was too upset, so I decided to go to my parents' house to vent and cool off. By the time I walked into their house, I was crying and told my dad what happened. He immediately put on his shoes and left for the restaurant to explain to the manager what I felt. The owner apologized to my dad, but he hadn't apologized to me. He told my dad that he was sorry that I felt that way but didn't say he was wrong."

Suzanne's story was repeated among Ability employees and many of them chose to boycott the restaurant after that episode. If this establishment was not okay for Jenn, it wasn't a place that they would patronize. Interestingly, that restaurant has since gone out of business.

CHRIS AND I had a similar episode. Before we discovered Bagelman, we had frequented another restaurant in Brookfield. They had good food and treated us well, so we returned there each week for lunch. Like Suzanne, Chris remembered our unfortunate episode there and although she didn't confide in me that day about her feelings, she later retold the story from her viewpoint.

"That day when we walked in, the waitress was kind of snarky. I don't know if she was having a bad day or what, but the first thing she said to us was, 'You are here all the time, you don't need a menu.'

"'No, we would like a menu,' I snarled back.

"Jenn was a little loud, but no more than usual. She was always excited and noisy until she sat down and had a soft drink in front of her, and then she'd quiet down. We were quickly seated in a booth in the main area. I don't know if it was because I was snarky back to the waitress when I said that we would like menus or what, but the woman who seated us went over to talk to the manager. The next thing I knew, he came over to us and said, 'Because of her noise level, would you mind moving to the back where the pool tables are?'

"'That's the smoking section, so no, we don't want to move back there,' I told him.

"'Well, I understand, but she is kind of loud.'

"'We are here every week; she is a human being. She's a person.'

"'I understand, I understand,' he told me before walking away.

"With that, Barb, you and I agreed we couldn't stay there. We had to leave because they wanted to put Jenn in the back, away from other patrons. I felt she was being very discriminated against. We'd been there every week for months, and suddenly her noise was an issue. They should have been used to her by now. When I got in the car, I was so upset I started to cry. I remember that you tried to calm me down and told me not to worry about it, but I couldn't let it go. Later I talked with Suzanne and other staff about it and decided it was time to find another place to go. I've never been back there since."

Chris continued, "I wanted to do something about this discrimination; it was not okay for this to happen. I was angry! When I started crying in the car that day, it wasn't because of embarrassment or humiliation, it was anger. I was mad and felt defeated; there was nothing I could do to protect Jenn from that kind of rejection. In the days that followed, I knew I needed to take some sort of action to advocate for Jenn. I contacted The Persons with Disabilities advocacy group in the state of Connecticut to find out what I could do. I also talked to our human resource department. They said word of mouth was the best way to handle it. If there had been Facebook at the time, I would have told everyone not to go to that restaurant as they don't like people with disabilities. They were lucky social media wasn't available then."

I knew that Jenn often created a spectacle in public places, and as much as I wanted things to be different, there was nothing I or anyone could do to make her behavior more appropriate. I came to expect that people at various businesses might be put off by her noises, and for us to be asked to leave, but I never got used to those kinds of rejections and neither did Chris or Suzanne.

For them, facing confrontations in restaurants was the most difficult and hurtful part of caring for Jenn. They wanted to be respectful of others in the community but still give Jenn the opportunity to be out like any other person.

I struggled with the thought of whose rights were being violated. Was it the other patrons' right to have a quiet environment for their dinner, or Jenn's right to partake in the restaurant's offerings? If other customers had more rights than Jenn, that would eliminate her from going on any extended outings.

I never had the right answer regarding Jenn's unsettling sounds and their effect on other patrons; possibly there was none. But one thing for sure, it made Bagelman all the more special to us. We loved this place for their food, tolerance, and warm welcome whenever we walked in the door.

"WHY DO YOU have a handicapped sticker in your car?" strangers would ask the girls in parking lots.

"She has no trouble walking, so why would you take this spot?" they'd ask.

True, Jenn could walk, but she had no awareness of the dangers in parking lots. It took a lot of training of both staff and Jenn to keep her safe around cars and roadways. She was strong and would quickly get out of her vehicle and race to a destination as soon as the car stopped, especially if it was a restaurant. Once she was free of the seatbelt, Jenn was in high gear to get going, and staff needed to safely direct her through the maze of parked cars and moving traffic.

We figured out that having her ride directly behind the driver was the quickest way to attend to her after parking. Once out of the car, managing this strong, racing adult through the lot was not for the timid or weak. The less time spent around traffic, the better. Handicapped spaces were closer to businesses and therefore an important safety factor for Jenn.

"There are other forms of disability besides ambulating issues that qualify a person for a handicap sticker," they'd say to the nosy stranger. Loud protests from Jenn for being held back from rushing out of the car was all the explanation the questioner needed before turning tail and leaving the scene.

WE KNEW BY now that Jenn could not read and had trouble interpreting images in photographs and matching them to similar objects. We tried many ways to communicate using visual instead of verbal cues, but nothing seemed to work.

Strangely enough though, Jenn recognized every restaurant we drove or walked by. She knew the golden arches—an old memory most likely—but she even recognized a little, local pizza parlor that had no logo to identify it as an eatery. Jenn did have an acute memory for all things related to food, so if she had eaten there before, she'd remember that valuable information. But sometimes we were not in a local area, and she was still able to tell which of the random storefronts were restaurants. How did she know? We were never able to figure it out. Sometimes there were things that Jenn did or didn't understand that we couldn't piece together and make sense of, but we tried. She was a puzzle that we constantly worked to solve.

MEDICAL APPOINTMENTS WERE always a challenge, and Jenn was in good hands when Chris and Suzanne accompanied her. In fact, they were often better at dealing with her in these situations than I was. They were stronger than me and this helped in managing her during these visits. I had total confidence in their judgment and advocacy for her. This trust was founded on the countless hours I'd spent working with these two young women and watching how they handled themselves and Jenn in many different situations through the years.

Sitting quietly in a doctor's waiting room until your name was called must have seemed pointless to Jenn. After what she determined was a long enough wait with nothing happening, she was ready to head for the door, but Chris or Suzanne would direct her back to her seat, which she loudly protested. They didn't take those outbursts as bad behavior; Jenn was just expressing what everyone feels when faced with a long wait in the doctor's office. The girls tried to keep Jenn as quiet as possible. But if the wait was too long, they decided her noise was a good lesson for the office in how to better manage their appointment scheduling.

"We gave up on keeping Jenn quiet and let the office hear her vocalizations. She was just expressing the general feeling of everyone in the waiting room."

Being tactile sensitive made any medical appointment quite hard for Jenn. Doctors had all kinds of touching requests, which only resulted in loud protests from her. Taking off her shoes was a serious enough offense—never mind someone touching what we came to know as her most sensitive area, her feet.

Trying to be ever so gentle, the doctors would approach Jenn doing the exact opposite of what they needed to do to examine her. When someone is tactile sensitive, the best method for contact is to not touch softly, but instead use a firm grip. Most doctors, however, were not interested in having family members or caregivers instruct them on how to go about their business. If a doctor gave a look that asked, *What did I do that made her so upset?* Chris, Suzanne, or I were more than happy to tell them what was wrong. But most of the time, they didn't ask for our opinions or suggestions and just got yelled at by Jenn. Some physicians took her inappropriate behaviors and noise in stride; others were more nervous and reluctant to proceed further.

If regular checkups were difficult for Jenn, imagine the problems associated with various medical screenings, especially a mammogram when Jenn turned thirty. All of us share in her discomfort with that test; Jenn was just more vocal in her reaction to it and very uncooperative with the process. Chris and Suzanne explained how they approached the situation.

"We came armed with a bag of M&Ms to help distract her, but not even those yummy treats convinced her to stand still for that uncomfortable position long enough for the technician to do her thing. We had to physically wedge her between us and the machine so she couldn't move as the test was performed."

How dedicated they were to manage that procedure and help their friend get the important screening. I don't think I would have been as resourceful or determined.

A food reward awaited Jenn once the torture was over, but I can't imagine what she must have thought was happening and why her friends would do a strange thing like this to her. Fortunately, she was never one to hold a grudge. Once released from the jaws of the mammogram machine and the human wedge, she acted like her happy self, ready to move on with her day.

Dental visits were equally invasive for Jenn, and an annual appointment for those checkups was guaranteed to be a bad day for her and a challenge for those who were with her. It was a struggle to get into her mouth to clean her teeth or check for cavities. We gave her Valium to calm her for a cleaning, but with head injuries, medications often work in a much different way than expected. Jenn was so energized after taking Valium that there was no chance things could go smoothly. As soon as a dental mirror was stuck into her mouth, she bit down on it and broke it to pieces. End of appointment! Time to figure out a different approach.

After several attempts with various providers, Chris talked with the pediatric dentist she took her kids to and he agreed to work with Jenn. A pediatric dentist knows that a great deal of patience is required, and his skill would be tested to the max with his new patient. Using food as a positive reinforcement for Jenn, she stayed cooperatively in the chair, and although she was loud in her objections, she let the doctor do his exam. Success—no broken mirrors or bitten fingers.

Fortunately, she had great teeth and few dental problems. Other than cleanings and exams, nothing else had to be dealt with.

HOSPITAL STAYS WERE also quite challenging for Jenn, as they required 24/7 coverage by either the staff, Mark, or me for her benefit and the safety of everyone at the hospital.

Jenn could not be left alone unsupervised in a room with tubes, machines, and other medical paraphernalia nearby. Given the opportunity, she would tamper with the buttons on the beeping IV monitor, pull tubes out of her arm, or even throw things across the room to get them out of her way. Picking the labels and decals off various machines or hardware was also a good form of entertainment for the bored patient.

Jenn was unable to communicate with nurses or doctors, so we had to be Jenn's voice and advocates. After her initial injury, she had corrective surgeries, infections, seizures, and a bad gallbladder to deal with, and each of these events required a hospital stay.

Jenn needed repeated nerve blocks for her right arm and hand to relieve pain and allow her greater range of motion. Those nerve block procedures were performed at Danbury Hospital. Our treating doctor, an anesthesiologist specializing in pain management, came to realize that getting her into the operating room required creative thinking to win the trust of his patient. He felt it would give her comfort to have me accompany her to the operating room. But he also didn't expect her to get on a gurney and be rolled down the corridors of the hospital. He let her walk on her own accord with him at her side.

Once Jenn was outfitted in her gown, shoe covers, and hair net, the doctor came into the waiting room to get us. He gently took Jenn by the arm, and together we walked with her down the hallway. Jenn seemed to know that this gentle man somehow helped to relieve her pain. She let him escort her into the bowels of the hospital to the operating room with its bright lights, monitors, and medical team that greeted her. She was compliant as nursing staff helped scoot her onto the operating table. I held her hand until the anesthesia took hold.

Danbury Hospital personnel became familiar with Jenn over the years and offered an abundance of kindness and understanding to their unique patient. Of course, there were always new members of the medical staff who would walk into the room unprepared for how to address a patient who was so disabled, especially a nonverbal one.

"Hello, Jenn, I am Doctor Smith, how are you doing today?" they'd say.

They'd seem more than a little confused when I told them Jenn was not able to communicate. Perplexed that she wouldn't understand their questions or be able to describe how she was feeling, and at a loss for how to proceed, they often continued with the standard routines. "What is your level of pain this morning?" or, "Can you take a deep breath for me?" That was never a productive scenario for Jenn or the doctor. I would have to intervene and say, "She doesn't understand your request to take a deep breath so just listen to her lungs as best you can and let it go at that. The nurses are doing a good job of monitoring her level of pain, and she seems more comfortable today."

There was always a learning curve for physicians when they were first introduced to Jenn. I liked to think that during their career, the lessons learned in dealing with her would resonate with them when it came to treating others with disabilities. Not all patients are textbook cases, and some skills must be learned in the field, not in medical school. Jenn gave the professionals who treated her the opportunity to work with a person with a compromised communication system. The experience doctors gained in working with Jenn would, we hoped, prove to be invaluable to them in the future.

Jenn served all of us well, including medical professionals, as a mentor for those who worked with people who had disabilities. By watching how she responded to Chris and Suzanne's gentle guidance and handling, the medical world where she received treatments learned how to lovingly interact with and encourage a patient to be cooperative so they could help her.

WE COULD TELL when Jenn was in pain, but it was difficult to determine where it was located. A grimace on her face or doubling over and groaning let us know that something was wrong. But what was the exact source of the problem: a stomachache, the reflex sympathetic dystrophy in her arm, gallbladder issues, a migraine, or was it something new and unknown to us? It always took lots of educated guessing to determine the cause.

There was a period of time when Jenn seemed uncomfortable while sitting and was hesitant to take a seat when we gestured for her to. Was she being stubborn or was there something wrong? "Maybe it's sciatica," Chris suggested thinking back to her past issue with it. An exam by her physical therapist confirmed our suspicions: sciatica. Along with some extra physical therapy exercises, the therapist recommended that we enroll her in the local gym to strengthen more muscles in her body.

From that point on, Jenn went to the gym twice a week for sessions with trainers who had expertise in treating people with disabilities. They had an interesting challenge when they introduced her to all the equipment, especially the treadmill. I loved watching their sessions to see how they managed a reluctant client on this machine. Facing forward and going at a slow speed was agreeable to Jenn, but they also expected her to use the treadmill standing sideways, doing a crossover with her legs in a grapevine movement. She could easily do this crossover stepping with one side of her body, but the other, weaker side was difficult.

Loud protests were directed at the trainers but that didn't seem to fluster them. They were not going to let Jenn scare them away from helping her do exercises that would reduce her sciatic pain. After several introductory sessions, Jenn quieted down a good amount but was never a fan of the sideways treadmill routine.

To get her to use the recumbent bike, I watched Chris or Suzanne move each of her feet in the circular motion needed to complete the full rotation of the pedals. She really didn't mind the biking segment of the session after she mastered the process and would cooperatively sit back and pedal until the timer went off. But after ten minutes when the alarm started beeping, she was off the machine in a flash.

I went along on many of those gym outings and was impressed with the loving care the trainers gave Jenn. It was also touching to see how they managed, after enduring a lot of screaming in her initial sessions, to get her to be compliant and even give them a smile or laugh during her workout. Through their patient encouragement, she slowly evolved into a happy and willing participant.

One thing for sure, those early gym sessions proved to be a great form of exercise for Chris and Suzanne. Working to get Jenn's legs to do the treadmill grapevine by physically moving her torso and limbs required a lot of stamina. Sitting on the floor holding Jenn's feet on the pedals of the bike and doing pedaling for her until she understood what was expected was also a real workout. I don't think Jenn ever broke a sweat during those sessions, but I am sure Chris and Suzanne did.

We continued Jenn's gym membership even after it was no longer needed for the sciatica problem. We wanted her to keep the physical gains that she had acquired during her treatment. She never experienced any sciatica problems after that, and we knew the regular exercise helped to keep her stronger and healthier. After a while, she began to view the gym outings in a positive way. She seemed to know where they were going when she was outfitted in her gym clothes and seemed excited to head out the door to a place where everyone was nice and welcoming to her. I could see that she was happy to be in a place that gave her positive reinforcement, even though she still didn't like the treadmill grapevine routine.

IN JENN'S EARLY years at Squire, Maria had worked extensively on taking her to movies, but it was still no simple matter when others tried this form of entertainment with her. Jenn had trouble sitting still for any length of time in those early days at Ability, and movies were no different. We thought that if she had popcorn, she would gladly stay seated while staff fed her one kernel of corn at a time. That worked to a point. What we saw was that Jenn wasn't looking at the screen at all—she was totally focused on the popcorn with her hand out, waiting for the next kernel to come her way.

As with most things we attempted with Jenn, we had as much to learn as she did. We had to know how to get her to do the things we wanted without making the situation more complicated and unmanageable. With the popcorn, we had set ourselves up for disaster. The only way we were going to get her absorbed in the film was to stop all food at the movies. We'd go to the theater but have to leave quickly because of a loud outburst from a very unhappy Jenn, who was being redirected away from the concession stands. After months of failed attempts, Jenn finally learned the new routine of walking past the food counter and we could take her to her seat and see the whole film without incident.

Once inside the theater, it was important that the correct kind of movie was being shown. The type of shows that would hold Jenn's interest were fast paced and action packed, or ones with lots of silliness. Chick Flicks and movies with long narratives were not something she understood, and she'd get restless at them. Movies designed for kids or action-packed dramas were a much better fit.

To Chris and Suzanne's way of thinking, if Jenn could now go to movies, why not a Broadway play? "Barb, we want to take Jenn to see Hairspray in New York. It's a loud and boisterous show that we think will keep Jenn's attention and mask any noises she makes," they told me.

"Give it a try," I encouraged them. "What's the worst that can happen—you'd have to leave the theater."

They made their plans and headed out to the Big Apple and their first Broadway show.

A few days after their return, I was all ears as they shared with me how it worked out.

"It went really well, and we had a blast," Chris happily reported.

Suzanne continued, "There isn't any food at the theaters, so we didn't have that issue. But there was one curious thing that happened, Jenn thought that when the audience started clapping after each song, it was her cue to stand up and leave. We had to redirect her to stay sitting, but that was fine. I don't think it was because she didn't like what was happening on stage, she must have just thought the applause was the end of the show. Then at the real ending, she seemed surprised when everyone was clapping and standing and now we expected her to get up too. It was kind of like, 'Why are we standing now when we couldn't before,'" Suzanne said with a laugh, "but when Jenn saw that we were leaving, she was excited to go."

"I can't wait to do it again," said Chris, "I love Broadway shows and if we can take Jenn, that would be perfect."

That opportunity came several months later when Chris saw that the Blue Man Group was performing in New York and thought this was the right kind of production for Jenn to see. After another brainstorming session, we worked out the details, and within weeks, they were again off to the city. I heard all about it after they returned.

"We got up early and met at Squire to get Jenn ready and pack her bag. She always gets excited to see her suitcase come out. She knows something fun is going to happen and probably can read the excitement in Chris and me too," Suzanne shared with me over lunch at Bagelman.

"It was cold, Barb, but we had Jenn bundled up like she was going to the Yukon. We drove to the station and caught the train into the city—so much easier than going by car." Chris added. "Jenn loves riding on the train. She laughs and looks out the window, waving at I don't know what, but she's happy."

"Once we got to the city and left the train, food concessions and bakeries were right there, and we had to walk past them to get to the exits," Suzanne continued. "This is the only problem with taking the train. Sometimes we stopped there for lunch, but most times we'd wait until we're out in the city to eat, which is what we did this time. Jenn got so excited to see all the food concessions we were passing that she tried to push her way to the nearest one. After getting her past it, she assumed the next place was where we were going and made a mad dash for it instead. The pushing, groaning, and redirecting continued until we reached the stairway leading to the outside ground level where there was no food to distract her."

Chris continued, "You know Jenn isn't a big fan of stairs, so she needed a little encouragement to do the climb up to street level, but she was more compliant once food wasn't in the picture."

"We hailed a taxi to bring us to the hotel where we checked in and dropped off our luggage," Suzanne said. At last, they were ready to begin taking in the city sights, and of course have the long-awaited lunch.

Jenn always seemed to be excited to be in the midst of all the city hubbub with her friends. Favorite stops like the M&M and Toys R Us stores offered ample entertainment for the three musketeers.

Street performers are a big part of the Times Square scene and add to the flavor of the experience. The Naked Cowboy was one such well-known character. Dressed in just his underwear—a pair of white briefs—and his cowboy hat, that performer played a guitar which was held so that from a distance he appeared to be wearing only his cowboy hat. He walked the streets, in clear view for shocked tourists to spot him, pull out their cameras, and hand over a few dollars for the privilege of taking his photo. "We couldn't believe we actually saw him, Barb," Suzanne excitedly told me. "Jenn couldn't have cared less, but Chris and I thought it was fun." This added to their adventure and certainly made for a juicy story when they returned home.

Time passed quickly for the three girls, and afternoon turned to evening. An Irish pub located right in the theater district seemed the perfect place to have dinner before heading to the show. The entrance for this restaurant was on the ground floor, but seating was in the upstairs level. More stairs! That was okay, though, because Jenn seemed to realize they were going to eat.

"She rushed as fast as she could up those two flights of stairs to the dining room," Chris said. "Once seated, we had a view that overlooked all the busyness of the city below, but Jenn didn't look at the view. She watched each tray of food that was brought into the dining room from the kitchen, hoping that this one was hers. As the trays came by their table, she would give a wave of welcome and loud gasp of excitement, only to watch it go past and on to another table."

New Yorkers have seen it all. They are rather numb when it comes to someone making unusual noises or exhibiting odd behaviors. "No one even gave Jenn a second glance as she did her routine of loudly reacting to each tray of food as it passed her by," Chris told me. Finally, the waiter stopped at her table and the long-awaited meal was served.

Once dinner was done and the bill paid, it was time for the girls to take to the city streets. The theater district is always busy, but in the hour before evening performances, crowds thicken, and pedestrians vie for space on the narrow walkways. Throngs of people line up in front of each theater.

"We each held on tightly to one of Jenn's hands and quickly wove our way through the mass of humanity," Chris explained.

Jenn was not one who liked to be rushed, pulled along, or have people bump into her. On the other hand, if she saw a restaurant ahead, she had no problem pushing past people and charging ahead like a running back for the NFL. But with no restaurant in sight, Chris and Suzanne had to grab on to her and plow ahead, undeterred by any resistance she gave.

Their story continued, "The good thing was that with the noise of the city all around us, no one could hear her loud protests as we pushed ahead and finally made it to our theater. Once inside, we climbed the stairs to our second-floor seats up in the balcony. Jenn didn't know exactly where we were going, but she knew we wouldn't lead her astray. She knew we had fun wherever we would take her. We put her in the seat between us, and she was in great spirits as we waited for the performance to begin."

Chris and Suzanne had come to expect that Jenn often got singled out of a crowd when they went places, but in a good way. They always loved to report back to me on those touching occasions. For example, when they went to Medieval Times for the dinner show, the knights, upon winning their round in various jousting competitions, presented a rose to some young lady in the audience. Every time the girls went, it was always Jenn who was handed the rose. She would willingly take the offering but didn't seem quite sure what to do with it. She would twirl it around for a while, and then give it a couple of shakes before discarding it on the table.

The Blue Man show proved to be no different. After taking their seats, a member of the stage crew came up to them and asked if Jenn would participate in their opening act after intermission. "Chris and I looked at each other and gave a snicker," Suzanne said with a laugh as she went on with her story. "'Sure,' I told him, 'but she might yell at you in the process.'"

No, I didn't think Jenn was picked because she was disabled. I also didn't think it was because she was pretty, as Suzanne and Chris liked to think was the reason. They told me Jenn was quietly sitting there as normally as any other person in the audience when he came up to them. My guess was that her specific seat was probably used for that act at every show. But for Chris and Suzanne, it made a better story when they said, "Of course they picked Jenn; it always happens."

Suzanne went on, "The crew guy explained that he needed Jenn to hand marshmallows to the Blue Man who would be standing behind her when the spotlight came on. He started to hand her a bag of marshmallows and of course Jenn got really excited and was eager to grab them from him."

"That's when I intervened," Chris added. "I told the crew member, 'Hmm, I'll take that.' There was no way Jenn wasn't going to eat those treats right away if she got her hands on them, and she was certainly not going to give them away to some stranger, even a blue one."

"We didn't really know what to expect at the end of intermission, and of course, Jenn had no idea that something unusual was going to happen," Suzanne remarked. "We were waiting for him to come. The lights flickered on and off signaling that intermission was about to end. But once the lights went out, it was still a little startling when the spotlight came on and instantly pointed directly at us. And there he was, this blue guy, standing right on the back of Jenn's chair. For Chris and me, it was a little alarming, never mind for Jenn—a blue person standing right above her as she looked behind to see what was going on. She was probably a little surprised to have him so physically close, and certainly not impressed when Chris started handing him all those tasty marshmallows which he began comically throwing at others in his troupe and also at various people in the audience. The whole act was bizarre from start to finish. They were blue people who didn't talk, took things, and threw stuff all around the theater. Jenn was probably wondering, what in the heck was going on here. It was weird from beginning to end, but really cool."

I often wondered if the adventures of Chris, Suzanne, and Jenn could possibly have been as silly and entertaining as the pictures they painted in their storytelling upon their return. But as they often reminded me, "You just can't make that kind of stuff up." It was always like that, the three of them finding humorous situations wherever they went. Or was it that unusual people and circumstances had a way of finding them? Stories like this gave me a way to enjoy my daughter as I never could have without the amazing adventurous spirit of Suzanne and Chris. It was clear they felt Jenn enhanced their adventures and experiences instead of detracting from them. She was the wind behind their sails—the one who pushed them toward the unexpected and surprising delights that came when the three of them were together.

Chapter 17

TRAVELS

Early in Jenn's recovery I recognized that I didn't have the energy or stamina to care for her more than a couple of days at a time. When we had her ourselves during weekends or holidays, I felt drained from the constant engagement that was required to keep her entertained and away from the refrigerator and cabinets. Although Mark and Amy were always on hand to help, I was the one responsible for her personal hygiene needs. Physically supporting her weight for bathing and toileting took its toll on my body, as did helping her dress and undress. It was more than I could handle.

Chris and Suzanne were more than two decades younger, so they could keep up with her far better than I could. But another more significant part was the absolute joy and fun they would bring to situations as they cared for her. Their expectations of her were different from mine. I was always striving for Jenn to behave like she did before her accident.

I found it physically and mentally exhausting to constantly be on guard watching her every move, redirecting her away from mischief and dealing with her unusual behaviors, especially in public. She was not the pre-accident daughter I'd so carefully raised until that fateful day in 1991. Chris and Suzanne had a far better attitude about caring for Jenn. They accepted her behaviors as just who she was. They often told me how fulfilling it was to watch Jenn having fun and to know they were having a positive impact on her life. They truly loved making her laugh and smile. Their dedication was a gift to our family and to Jenn.

I wanted to be as upbeat as they were when I cared for Jenn, but I was battling my own scars of loss and despair from her accident. It was hard for me to be funny or silly, to look beyond the damage I could see in my daughter, no matter how hard I tried. Like them, I too loved when she laughed and smiled, but they were far better at accomplishing this task with her than I ever could be. I came to accept the reality that in order for us to include Jenn in any vacation or travel with us, we needed help. Fortunately, Suzanne and Chris were more than willing to work with us on this matter.

Traveling beyond the local area was a challenge Chris and Suzanne looked forward to and were excited about, but I recognized the many hurdles they had to navigate for a successful trip. I loved that they not only took on the responsibility of planning and logistics for these trips but were also willing to take time away from their families in order to give Jenn the opportunity to adventure to new places.

Soon after joining our team in 2002, Suzanne was initiated into the process of vacationing with Jenn when she and Chris planned a trip to Disney World where Mark and I met up with them. "Barb, it was the most memorable trip I took with Jenn," Suzanne reminisced. "Seeing the ecstatic look on Jenn's face as she walked up the path to Cinderella's Castle and suddenly spotted you and Mark standing there was a deeply touching moment for me—one I will never forget."

I remembered that exact moment myself—the surprised look on Jenn's face as though she could hardly believe her eyes. She had traveled a great distance and, out of nowhere, her mom and dad appeared. There was no way to convey to her ahead of time that we would be meeting her at Disney. She couldn't anticipate that we had flown in on our own and would be standing in front of Cinderella's Castle waiting to join in her adventure. Once she spotted us, a big smile appeared on her face and, with loud squeals of delight, she rushed up to give both of us a hug. It was a magical moment, and Suzanne got teary-eyed as she watched it unfold. My eyes misted up as well with the warm and touching exchange of raw emotion expressed by our daughter who lacked words but whose loving message of joy was clear.

The five of us stayed at the Caribbean Beach Resort in Disney. We loved the island theme and the steel drum music that played over the loudspeakers throughout the grounds. All of us felt we had escaped to paradise. Disney didn't disappoint in entertaining us beyond our lodging area either.

We enjoyed most of the usual attractions throughout Disney, and all of them seemed to totally delight our daughter. She particularly liked the Mad Hatter's teacups and was much more tolerant of the spinning than we were. After each of us had taken her on this ride several times, we'd had enough, and it was time to head off to a less-nauseating activity.

Pre-accident, Jenn loved carnival rides and that still held true. Although she had an uneven gait on terra firma, she seemed to easily tolerate the spinning, twisting motion of those kinds of rides.

Early in her rehab, Jenn's occupational therapist suggested that we take her on carousels or swings, as it was a helpful treatment for her to experience different types of motion. She explained that studies showed that rolling and spinning were necessary for the proper development of a child's brain. Because Jenn was relearning how to use her body, the theory was that her brain might need the same stimulation as a young child's. I don't know if experiencing these rides helped her physically or mentally, but she did love them, and maybe, just maybe, they helped.

CHRIS'S FAVORITE BUT scariest trip with Jenn was in 2004, thirteen years after the accident, when she and Suzanne took Jenn to Bermuda. As she explained to me, "I was always nervous when we had to fly with Jenn. If we went by car and something went wrong, we could just turn around and go home. But if we were flying, it wasn't as easy to change plans. By going to Bermuda, not only were we going by plane, we were going out of the country!" But being adventuresome, she wanted to give it a try and depended on her resourcefulness to take care of anything that might go amiss.

Passports in hand, the girls set off for an island vacation in paradise. "We were pleasantly surprised and impressed with being able to pull off boarding, and the flight was easy as was Bermuda customs," Chris said. "I started to feel that this plan just might work after getting past all those hurdles. Once we got to our hotel, it really did begin to feel like a vacation because I noticed the kind way everyone acted toward Jenn. It was different than in the States, and I loved it."

Chris and Suzanne were used to being on guard to keep Jenn quiet when out in public. This tension was not present in Bermuda. "No one gave us odd looks when Jenn made her noises, and we were never turned away from any establishments. In fact, we were welcomed and shown much kindness and appreciation for our business," Chris reported. "For me, this was the most relaxing of all the outings we ever took together."

When they told me about their trip, I sensed they were able to kick back and enjoy the pristine island with its colorful foliage, world-class beaches, quaint towns, and wonderful inhabitants.

Like everyone who travels to Bermuda, Chris and Suzanne were excited to hit the beaches and partake in the true island experience of sand and warm tropical water. The clear ocean waves that lapped the shore at Horseshoe Bay were easily entered without the shock that comes when wading into the frigid water's edge of the Jersey shore. "With Chris on one side and me on the other, we had no problem getting Jenn to go into the water. She loved it," Suzanne said. "We went out up to our chests and Jenn was doing great, but Chris wasn't too thrilled," she added, chuckling.

Chris preferred pools to lakes and oceans. "Things live in the ocean," Chris said. "It was even worse in Bermuda. You could see things because the water was so clear. Fish were all around our legs, and that freaked me out," she said with a laugh.

Suzanne picked up the story. "So poor Chris was stuck with us out in the water. She was totally focused on watching all those colorful tropical fish swimming around us like we were a coral reef. Every time a fish got close to her, she would jump and scream. Of course, Jenn thought Chris's reactions were hysterical, and we laughed so hard we cried as we waited for Chris's next scream. Some of the fish were pretty big, and that sent Chris into hysterics. The more Chris reacted to the fish, the more Jenn and I cracked up."

At that point in the story, I said, "What a champion friend you are to experience what was for you a nightmare situation, and you hung in there for Jenn."

"Believe me, I wouldn't do it for anyone else," Chris quickly pointed out.

Island life was slow paced, and for Chris and Suzanne, who were used to very busy schedules, that was a special time to live in the moment and do whatever came along. "Our only time constraints were those set by empty stomachs or when exhaustion told us it was time for sleep. It was a freedom we'd seldom experienced before, and it set that trip apart from all others," Chris told me.

They were concerned about how they'd gain reentry into the States when it was time to return. Upon entering the US, customs agents ask all adults questions to establish if you are really who you say you are. "When it was our turn," Chris explained, "I told the agent that he could ask Jenn all the questions he wanted, but she was nonverbal and wasn't going to answer. It must have been pretty apparent to him that Jenn was special. He was very understanding and after a few friendly comments, welcomed the three of us back home." She laughed as she added, "I was thinking, what if I have to call Barb and say, 'Sorry, we had to leave Jenn in Bermuda.' Better yet, 'The three of us have to stay in Bermuda'—that wouldn't have been so bad; in fact, that would have really been okay."

I felt as if I'd been there with them as I heard the stories. It filled my heart with joy that Jenn and her good friends, Chris and Suzanne, could have such a grand time.

AS JENN'S CAREGIVERS expanded their travels to more exotic and interesting places, I understood they too were having a great time. It was a huge perk for Maria and later for Chris and Suzanne to have these opportunities. But that was a good thing. It was important for the staff to be excited about new adventures they could take with Jenn. The more hype and excitement that was injected into their work, the more refreshed and positive they would be in the long-term to carry them through the rough parts of caring for my daughter. It was important for her workers not to feel stuck in a repetitive routine and become bored with the day-to-day doldrums of giving personal care to a client. Jenn's happiness depended upon it.

Jenn had fun doing local things with her friends, but when Chris and Suzanne were excited about a new adventure, Jenn picked up on that energy, and she resonated to their enthusiasm.

These travels were a significant part of my plan to keep staff engaged in making life a wonderful journey for my daughter—one filled with laughter, new horizons, and variations from daily routines. It was amazing to watch my plan successfully unfold and become a reality for Jenn.

THE MOST UNUSUAL trip for the girls was in 2005 when they went to Parsons, Kansas, where Mark and I, along with several members of my family, would be visiting for a few days. I wanted Jenn to be there too. Chris and Suzanne volunteered to bring her, as they were up for the adventure—they'd never been to the Midwest.

Mark and I traveled to Kansas separately from the three girls, so they had to fill me in on their experience once they arrived at Parsons. "As soon as we drove out of the Tulsa airport, we saw what a unique landscape it was. There were endless fields of flat farmland dotted by oil wells and cattle grazing in the late afternoon sun. Toto, I think we *are* in Kansas, was the thought Chris and I shared as we drove across the plains. The hour-and-a-half drive from Tulsa to Parsons was an eye-opener for us," Suzanne excitedly told me.

Chris added, "I felt nervous going through the little towns because you had warned us how the speed limit would go from fifty to twenty in a heartbeat, and a local sheriff could be hiding anywhere to pounce on unsuspecting travelers like us. I didn't want to end up in a small-town jail for speeding. As we traveled down the road, we didn't see any signs of civilization for a long time. Then some shopping centers and stores would appear, only to quickly fade into nothingness again. There were lots of small back roads and not many highways, whereas in the Northeast there are major roads everywhere."

Suzanne had a similar viewpoint: "It was literally fields and tumbleweeds as far as the eye could see—open areas of nothing. When we got into Parsons, it was adorable and clean, a tiny one-stoplight, Midwest town like you read about in books. We'd never seen anything like it. I loved it! I could live there in a heartbeat—I think. It's so busy in the Northeast."

Their destination was my sister's house where they met her and her husband, my niece's family, and a cousin and her husband who had driven up in their RV rig from Louisiana.

My eighty-four-year-old father, Les, resided in the local assisted living facility and would also be part of the gathering.

After arriving, the girls easily fit in with the family waiting to welcome them into my sister's small ranch-style home, typical of residences there. Jenn was bubbly and seemed excited to be in the midst of so many friendly people. I don't know if she recognized any of the Kansas folks as her own kin, but she made her loud happy screams of delight as each of them came up to embrace her.

As evening came, it was time to call it a day. My sister's house couldn't accommodate all the additional guests who had come for the reunion, so Chris, Suzanne, Jenn, Mark, and I all stayed at the local motel on the edge of town.

There was no breakfast provided by the motel, so each morning we went to the Breakfast Nook downtown where we met my father, who went there for breakfast every morning.

When he walked in the door, the person behind the counter would always greet him with, "Good morning, Les, will it be the usual today?"

For my dad, the first component of any meal was the requisite cup of coffee with six heaping teaspoons of sugar and enough milk added to bring it to a light caramel color. Breakfast included a bowl of Wheaties with an ample amount of milk to totally submerge the cereal flakes that he would top off with more sugar, lots of sugar. As hard as it might be to understand, all this caloric intake did nothing to increase the man's waistline. He was thin as a rail his whole life and would continue to be for his remaining days.

For the rest of us, we loved the Breakfast Nook's hot cinnamon rolls, and their pancakes were world-class. The cozy 1940s atmosphere of this small café magically made us feel like we were in another time and place.

Chatter was lighthearted and constant as we enjoyed our sumptuous breakfast fare, with Jenn smiling and nodding, as this was her way of contributing to the conversation going on all around the table. Those would be some of the last breakfasts I'd share with my dad, and I can't think of a more endearing place to have made such sweet memories.

I don't remember ever going back to Kansas in the summer without having a tornado threat, and that time was no different. As we lightheartedly chatted throughout the afternoon with a hot game of Pictionary in progress, clouds began to build up outside, and the weather channel on the living room television started blasting alerts of an approaching storm system. Chris and Suzanne couldn't believe what was happening. "Oh my gosh, we *are* in Kansas!" they said.

The girls had heard stories of how the little downtown of Parsons had been flattened only four years earlier by a tornado, so all of us took this warning seriously. The TV weather alert began beeping, and a loud blare sounded from the local storm warning system my sister had installed in her house. Alarms were going off everywhere!

Our only shelter was located under the house, a crawl space four feet high with a dirt floor that extended under the foundation with an access hole in the garage floor. One had to crawl through the hole on all fours to enter the shelter. The space had been readied for emergencies, so necessities like bottled water, nonperishable food, a battery-operated radio, flashlights, and blankets were all in place.

Tornadoes were in the area and we were under a "watch" alert, a time to be vigilant and ready to seek shelter. We were not yet at the "warning" level, but if that happened, we would need to quickly head to the crawl space.

Rather than being alarmed by all the loud alerts going off in my sister's house, Jenn seemed to think it was all quite funny. She added to the noise level with her high-pitched screeches of excitement as she walked around the house giving everyone arm squeezes and over-the-top loud laughs as though we were having a party and she was in the mood to celebrate.

After about an hour of beeps, alarms, and rattled nerves, the threatening part of the storm dissipated before it got to Parsons. We all lived to see another day, and the rest of the visit went without any more weather interruptions.

It's fair to say that Chris and Suzanne had a true Kansas experience during that visit. With the storm moving on to locations well beyond Parsons, all the excitement ended up just making for an interesting tale to spin when they returned home to their families in Connecticut.

CHRIS AND SUZANNE'S adventures with Jenn did a great deal to expand my ideas of what could and should be done with a person who had disabilities. To quote Oliver Wendell Holmes, Jr., "A man's mind, stretched by new ideas, may never return to its original dimensions." In hearing the girls' stories, my mind was forever broadened, and I knew that Jenn's world was limited only by our imaginations.

Chapter 18

THE WEDDING

Eleven years after Jenn's accident, our Amy was all grown up. After attending college at Boston University and then graduate school, majoring in speech–language pathology at Massachusetts General Hospital, she stayed in Boston and began working in a nearby school district. A chance encounter in the populous sprawl of this big city would become a big life changer for her. It was one of those serendipitous moments when the paths of two young adults crossed, unaware that they would soon begin a relationship and fall in love. Jeff was a tall, handsome guy riding on the Boston T—the subway—with his eye on a cute, petite girl chatting away across the aisle from him.

Months after this encounter and well into dating Amy, Jeff told me the story of how he had first met her and what his thoughts were then. "Amy was totally unaware that the conversation she was having on the T that day caught my ear when she mentioned the name 'Pia,' a friend she would be meeting up with later that evening. It's not that common a name, and my childhood friend by that name lived in Boston. I thought, it just had to be the same person."

Jeff saw an opportunity to have his friend introduce him to the interesting girl he'd spotted on the subway. "Her fellow passenger referred to her as Amy, so I knew her first name. I called Pia as soon as I got home and asked if she knew a girl by that name. I described her as petite, beautiful, and funny, and said I'd like to meet her. She knew exactly who I was describing.

"'Yes, I know her, Jeff, but the timing isn't good. She just broke up with her boyfriend, and I think it's too soon to introduce her to someone else,' Pia told me."

But as luck would have it, he didn't have to wait for an introduction. A group of mutual friends happened to meet for dinner a few days later at a local restaurant. Amy and Jeff were both there.

"I was stuck at the opposite end of the table, so I couldn't catch Amy's attention, but I was determined not to let my chance to meet this girl slip away. Once everyone had finished their meal, I maneuvered into position to strike up a conversation with her and then had the chance to walk her home. Along the way, she gave me her phone number, and we made plans to meet again in a few days for dinner.

"Our first date turned out to be a great evening of conversation at a local pub. I quickly realized that Amy was a lot more than just a pretty face. She was smart but humble. I could tell she had a big heart and loved people. There was also an energy about her when she talked that captivated me. I knew I was interested in discovering more about her and spending more time with her."

After their successful first date, Amy and Jeff found every opportunity to be together as often as possible in spite of their busy schedules. Within a few months, Jeff, always one to get right to the point, asked Amy, "Do I stand a chance with you, or should I move on?" Fortunately for them both, Amy replied that he did stand a chance, and a new romance took flight in June of 2001.

Over the course of the next year, as I got to know Jeff better, and he became more familiar with our family, I was curious about what his thoughts were when Amy told him about Jenn, and what it was like to meet her for the first time.

"My initial response to Amy's description of her sister must have seemed odd to her when I look back on it," he explained. "I thought Jenn's injury was probably the same thing as the concussions I'd seen athletes get all the time, and they seemed to do fine after missing a couple of games. Amy had to set me straight. 'No, it's bad, Jeff, and Jenn has many disabilities. My sister was beautiful and fun before her accident. Now, it's like someone else is walking around in her body.'

"As Amy explained her sister's injury in more detail to me, I realized her condition was far beyond anything I'd known. I was the same age as Jenn, so I had a hard time imagining a life turned upside down so radically.

"The first time I met Jenn was when Amy and I were driving to New Jersey from Boston for the Thanksgiving holiday. Amy wanted to stop in Danbury, Connecticut to see Chris and Jenn. Chuck's Steak House was just off Interstate 84, a great location to meet for lunch before we continued on to New Jersey."

"Did Amy prep you before you got to Chuck's, and were you nervous to meet Jenn after hearing about her disabilities?" I asked.

He took a moment to collect his thoughts, and his blue eyes looked off into the distance as he pondered his answer.

"Amy didn't really prep me. She just said, 'Jenn can walk, but she can't talk.' She probably told me that Jenn might be loud, but I was used to being around pretty loud people. I didn't know what to expect, but I wasn't shocked by any of it. For me, it was like meeting anyone else. Unfortunately, I couldn't have a conversation with Jenn, but I tried to make eye contact with her. I watched Amy for cues on how to act around her sister and emulated whatever she did. I would say that's how I based all my interactions with Jenn—to follow Amy's lead." With a chuckle, he added, "The system of following Amy's lead seems to work out for most things in my life."

"What was your first impression of Jenn?"

He was quick to respond, "Her noises were certainly different from most people's. I just never gave them a second thought. We were eating lunch and having a good time. I'm sure that for Suzanne, Chris, you, Mark, and Amy, her noises were more difficult to be around. For me, I was new to the situation, and spending time around her wasn't a challenge. It was interesting to meet a person who'd suffered such a dramatic change in her life and yet could be so happy and engaging with her sister and Chris. Jenn was using all kinds of body language and facial expressions to show how thrilled she was to see Amy. Excitement just seemed to ooze out of her, and she had a hard time holding it in. Although she was a bit too loud, how can you fault a person who has no other way to show you how happy they are to see you?"

Jeff further explained how he'd tried to piece together an image of Jenn pre-accident. "That was the Jenn who had me the most curious. Trying to understand the sister Amy grew up with and imagining the loss Amy must have felt was hard for me to wrap my mind around. All of us understand that at some point we must face the sickness and loss of elderly family members, however hard that may be. But when I thought of how a young teen would handle the tragic situation that Amy endured while she was in middle school, I was amazed at her strength. She not only survived the ordeal but thrived in spite of it, as evidenced by her academic accomplishments, her upbeat and positive nature, and the loving way she interacts with all those around her. I'm thankful that she used those harsh life lessons to build her character. I think it must have given her the determination to meet challenges head on and still retain the softer, kind person inside who freely opens her heart to accept everyone."

I was deeply touched by how much he appreciated Amy's beautiful nature, and that he understood and respected the many challenges she'd faced as a result of her sister's injury.

He continued, "I don't ask Amy too many questions about the accident. I'm afraid to stir up those sad and depressing memories. I'm protective of her feelings and emotions and steer away from making her look back and dig into the past."

Mark and I had also avoided talking about the past with Amy. Had we left her to process all her feelings about the accident on her own and, in so doing, done her an injustice? Amy's personality seemed so whole and complete. All of us were cautious about delving into a topic that might bring her back to a dark place.

AFTER THE INITIAL lunch with Chris and Jenn, Jeff didn't meet the rest of the Danbury crew until the following summer when he came to the beach house in Ocean City,

New Jersey for Jenn's annual vacation with staff and family. Here he had his first true glimpse into the web of relationships within our family.

Everyone was crowded into a small seaside cottage with bedrooms shared by members of the same gender. Jeff was housed with Chris's boys, Ian and Aaron who, at five years old, seemed to think that Jeff was just a big kid whose sole purpose in being there was to play with them—they were constantly vying for his attention. Games of catch and rowdy horseplay made him a big hit with the boys. All the while, Chris and Suzanne were carefully scrutinizing Amy's beau to see if this guy showed any promise as a family man. They had Amy's best interests in mind and carefully scouted out how he handled himself with their children. After they'd watched him over several days sharing laughs and fun with all the young ones in our group, we all talked it over and decided he was a pretty good catch. Well done, Jeff, you passed muster with the girls.

The vacation occurred early in the relationship, and all of us wanted the couple to take their time, but some important tests had been passed. Jeff was kind and understanding toward Jenn and didn't seem to be put off by her outbursts or behaviors. He seemed extremely attentive to Amy and was great around kids. Time was all that was needed for the new couple to grow and develop their relationship. It was no surprise to any of us when, three years later, they made plans to walk down the aisle and make a permanent commitment to each other.

In the summer of 2004, wedding preparations were quickly coming together for Amy and Jeff. Although Jenn was not capable of serving as the maid of honor or bridesmaid, Amy wanted her to look the part and have a matching bridesmaid gown and accessories.

Mark and I went to Danbury where we could take Jenn to the local David's Bridal Shop and have her fitted for a gown. Chris and Suzanne were excited to be part of the process and eager to help get Jenn dressed and undressed in the changing room. We knew she wasn't going to be thrilled at the idea of taking off her clothes and putting others on—she hated doing that. But Chris, Suzanne, Mark and I were determined to make it fun and special for her by being a bit over-the-top on our reactions to any silliness we could muster.

As expected, Jenn's verbalizations from the changing room left little doubt to Mark and me as we waited just outside that she was not a happy camper. Once Chris and Suzanne had her in the gown, they brought her out from the changing room and helped her up on the foot-high platform where the three-sided mirrors allowed all of us to see the beautiful reflection of our Jenn all dressed up and glowing in her full-length evening gown. We were surprised to witness a notable change in her demeanor. She'd transformed into a giddy but elegant young woman who seemed pleased with what she saw in the mirror. She appeared to be mesmerized by her image. Leaning closer to the mirror, she touched the fabric of her dress as if to study the soft texture of the satin as she ran her fingers up and down the bodice. Lifting the hem ever so slightly, she flipped the skirt as though she were dancing, or maybe she enjoyed seeing the movement of the material as it swept back and forth across her legs. She kept giving little waves to Mark and me as well as Suzanne and Chris as if to say, *Look at my dress—it's amazing*.

Pre-accident Jenn was thrilled the first time she wore an evening gown to go to the prom with her boyfriend, Greg. I saw that same glee and twinkle in her eye as she turned first in one direction and then the other in front of the mirrors at the bridal shop. As I watched her, tears of melancholy and joy came to my eyes. To see such happiness in my daughter was emotionally overwhelming. She made the simple act of dressing up and our making a big fuss about how she looked into an amazing few priceless moments at the bridal shop. I held that memory in my heart as a powerful reminder that joy could reach into the depths of my despair, touch me, and bring me to a better place.

As much as Chris, Suzanne, Mark, and I loved that Jenn was enjoying herself as she looked at her image in the mirrors, it was challenging for the person trying to pin her gown for the needed alterations. Standing still was not one of Jenn's better skills, and many of the carefully placed pins had to be redone, but the patient tailor finally got things right.

WHEN THE BIG day for Amy's wedding came, many of Jenn's current and previous staff, along with their spouses, were invited guests. All of them knew us and our family well and had been an integral part of Amy's life. But for some of Jeff's family and friends, this was their first introduction to Jenn.

Although everyone on the guest list knew that Amy's sister was somehow disabled from an accident, not everyone had met her or fully understood her condition. Amy decided to use a fun photograph of her and Jenn together in Boston (a trip shared with Maria, one of Jenn's first caregivers), along with a tastefully written message describing Ability Beyond Disability's role in her sister's life. The framed letter was placed next to the guest book for all to see upon their entrance to the wedding venue. It served as the guests' introduction to Jenn, and an explanation saying in lieu of party favors, the bride and groom would make a donation to this organization.

The wedding was held at a local catering facility in a town near Washingtonville. The ballroom overlooked a golf course with lush greenery extending to the sweeping mountain range in the distance. In the midst of this beautiful setting, Amy and Jeff exchanged their wedding vows and the guests welcomed the new Mr. and Mrs. O'Connor into the loving folds of family and friends. Both bride and groom glowed as they walked back down the aisle with Jeff's arm lovingly wrapped around Amy's waist.

Perfect July weather gave all the wedding guests ample opportunity to enjoy the outdoor balcony throughout the afternoon and evening. This setting also proved to be beautifully scenic for the many photo ops for guests, the wedding party, and our family: Jenn, Mark, Amy, me, and our newest member, Jeff. With smiles glowing in reflection of our inner joy, ours was the picture of a perfect family. In our wedding finery, facing the camera, we gave no evidence of what we had suffered over the past thirteen years. The day was not to be marred with sadness or pain. We were happy to be together and celebrating a special couple on their wedding day.

And with that, the party began! I don't think I've ever experienced a more energized group of people who loved to dance. With everyone on their feet, Jenn was right in the middle of the celebration. A conga line quickly formed and wove its way around the room picking up any stragglers who did not join on their own. Waving napkins as props for the dance, the room exploded with the beat of the music and thunderous laughter of party guests. Then, it was on to the next song and new moves were taken up where the conga line had been.

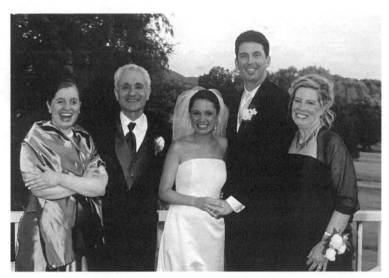

Amy and Jeff's wedding. Left to right: Jenn, Mark, Amy, Jeff, Barbara

At the close of the evening's festivities, we enjoyed the most memorable dance. "New York, New York" began playing and everyone locked arm-in-arm in a big circle, kicked legs like the Rockettes, and sang along with the lyrics. As I looked over and saw Jenn with Amy, Jeff, and all the wedding guests celebrating in a joyful way, I was struck by how our family had come so far after a horrific tragedy. We could be happy. We celebrated special occasions. We embraced life and were thankful that we still had each other, and our circle of family had grown to include Jeff's people and the Connecticut folks that Jenn had brought into our lives.

As the day and evening unfolded, and Jeff and Amy began their new life as a married couple, I looked around and marveled at the wonder of so many people who had been brought together: some by chance, some by bloodline, but all rejoicing for the bride and groom.

FAST FORWARD TWO years to 2006, and our young couple was expecting their first baby. Chris and Suzanne may have been as excited as Amy and Jeff by this welcome news. Amy and Jeff had been living and working in San Francisco, but once Amy was pregnant, they returned to the East Coast and settled in Moorestown, New Jersey. It was important to Amy that she be close to family and friends by the time children were born.

As soon as Chris and Suzanne heard that Amy and Jeff were expecting, they asked if they could plan a baby shower for Jenn to give for her sister. For this expenditure, I had to consult with the bank trustees to be sure they were on board with allowing Jenn's funds to be used in this way.

"Not so fast," said the banking cotrustee. "The money will not be spent for Jenn's benefit, but for Amy's." I needed to educate the new banking official who was overseeing Jenn's trust.

"Under any normal circumstances, a sister would give a baby shower for her sibling. There is no reason why a person who is disabled shouldn't be able to do the same thing," I went on to explain. "Don't you see all the fun Jenn will have going shopping for decorations, invitations, paperware, and all things related to giving a baby shower? The event will be held at Amy's home, so it isn't going to be an extravagant affair. It will be small and certainly isn't going to jeopardize the trust's stability."

She finally agreed that we had a good argument to present to the Surrogate's Court if we were questioned, and she gave me a green light for the party plan to proceed.

Chris, Suzanne, and Jenn did an amazing job with the party. As expected, Jenn had a blast sticking up streamers with lots of tape, putting balloons on the walls, setting up party ware, and basking in the excitement as they prepared for the joyful event. Laughs and camaraderie abounded as the three friends worked to make everything just right. The shower was a big success, and with the many generous gifts from guests, Amy was well prepared for motherhood. A few weeks later, she delivered a beautiful baby boy—Ryan.

AS A NEW grandmother, I found that instead of my thoughts being totally consumed with Jenn's care, I spent a lot of time thinking about the beautiful gift Amy and Jeff brought into my life. I traveled to New Jersey to help Amy with baby Ryan at every opportunity. Knowing that Jenn was in good hands with Chris and Suzanne, I felt the liberty to freely spend precious moments with my other daughter and grandson. My motherly instincts came to the surface as I held this tiny infant. I reminisced about the days when I held my own baby daughters and dreamed of all that life would hold for them. For Amy, those dreams had come true, but for Jenn they had been shattered. Although I recognized this harsh reality, Ryan brought such joy into my life that I didn't dwell on the dark thoughts of Jenn's tragedy as much as I had in the past. A new light was shining in the darkness of my mind as I gazed into the face of the sleeping bundle I held close to my heart.

Chapter 19

SPECIAL OCCASIONS

Could Jenn anticipate when a special occasion was on the horizon? When she got dressed up for Amy's wedding, did she know where she was going? When she saw her sister pregnant with Ryan, did she know it meant Amy was going to have a baby? Did memories from before or after the accident give her clues that a holiday was coming when she helped both the Benz and Boisvert families decorate their Christmas tree? There was no way to know how Jenn perceived all this—our questions would remain unanswered. We knew that Jenn fed off the body language of those around her, and if there was excitement in the air, she more than matched our energy with a loud and boisterous hype that demonstrated she knew something fun was in the works.

ONE SPECIAL OCCASION that happened every year and was right up Jenn's alley was Super Bowl Sunday. Was she into football either before or after her accident? No, but that wasn't what made it special for Jenn—it was how Suzanne's husband, Scott, celebrated the occasion with Jenn at his side.

Super Bowl Sunday was always a big deal at the Benz house. Wings, chips, and dips were required for Scott and the friends who came over for the game. Suzanne told me stories about the fun she and Jenn had preparing food all day, and how Jenn's excitement escalated as she waited to partake in all the yummy edibles.

"Guess who's right in the middle of the party when the game begins—Jenn," Suzanne explained. "Scott and his friends expect her, and they wouldn't have it any other way. Besides the food, I also think she's entertained watching the guys hollering and jumping up and down when their team scores a touchdown. I have to agree, they are pretty funny. Jenn has no interest in the TV or game—she just watches the food and the silly antics of Scott and his friends. They probably use as much energy watching the game as the players do on the field."

Suzanne also recounted Scott's video game nights. "When his buddies come over to hang out and play games, Jenn is right in there with them. It's the same entertainment for her as Super Bowl Sunday: finger foods, men jumping around, yelling, laughing, and acting ridiculously funny."

It was heartwarming for me to hear Suzanne's stories about Scott and Jenn. They shared a special bond of similar interests: food, laughing, silliness, and friendship. It was one more piece of a truly meaningful life that Suzanne and Christine brought into Jenn's otherwise handicapped world.

FOUR YEARS AFTER Amy's wedding, one of Jenn's previous caregivers, a delightful girl named Sue, wanted Jenn to be at her destination wedding in Florida. Sue had met Craig, her husband-to-be, at the Squire group home while working for Jenn. She told us it was a high priority for her to have Jenn there along with Chris, Suzanne, Mark, and me. We were all more than glad to oblige, and we flew down to The Don Caesar resort in St. Petersburg for the celebration.

In the warm Florida sunshine, surrounded by lush tropical plantings in the resort's garden, we all witnessed Sue and Craig's union. Jenn wore a green satin dress and glowed with the joy of having so many of her people there on a special day.

After the nuptials, a reception with dancing had Jenn out on the floor with all the other partygoers. Encouragement from Chris and Suzanne to shake her booty and move her body to the beat had Jenn hamming it up and adding her own special moves to the music. The room was rocking with loud rhythms from the DJ, and the party was in full swing with Jenn right in the middle. I couldn't help but be overjoyed and deeply touched to see my daughter included in the energetic celebration and, most importantly, accepted for who she was—disabilities and all. She was fully engrossed in the music and living it up with all the people who loved her and were thrilled in having her join in the fun.

There was also plenty of food, Jenn's favorite part of any gathering. From start to finish, the wedding celebration was a truly perfect day in paradise that continued on well into the evening.

We purposely added an extra day at the resort, as did many other wedding guests, to enjoy the pool, beautiful Florida weather, and extended time with family and friends.

The pool must have looked inviting to Jenn as she let us easily guide her down the ladder to step into the water. With assistance from us to help her keep her balance, Jenn cautiously tested the water temperature with her toe before going in. She loved to be in warm water as it seemed to soothe her tight muscles.

While in the pool, an old memory must have popped into Jenn's head—she attempted to swim. In waist-deep water, Chris and Suzanne lifted her into a floating position and without any direction or encouragement, she began to move her arms in the perfect motion of a crawl.

"Barb, look, she's trying to swim," an excited Chris yelled to me.

"Keep going Jenn, you're doing great," Suzanne encouraged.

Because of her compromised arm and leg, Jenn couldn't propel herself forward and maintain a floating position without Chris and Suzanne supporting her. But just seeing her try something that she was able to do pre-accident was a special moment for all of us.

Even if Jenn was unable to swim, that didn't diminish the fun she had splashing around in the water with all of us. She wasn't a big fan of being on the receiving end of a splash but laughed hard when she doused anyone who came within reach. We observed her relaxed posture and understood how therapeutic the pool was for her, but at some point we had to get out. Jenn had been slow to enter the pool but totally resistant to leaving her warm wet sanctuary, even if all the rest of us were shriveled up like prunes from being in the water too long.

"Jenn, you want a snack?" Chris asked as she held out some Goldfish crackers. With that inducement, Jenn couldn't get out quickly enough.

Once out of the pool, basking in the sun on the cushioned lounge chair wasn't so bad either. The day was spent around the pool, with all the wedding guests enjoying old stories and making new memories. This might have been the happiest any of us had seen Jenn since her accident. She smiled, laughed, squeezed arms, and head bumped everyone continuously over the long weekend. Her happiness couldn't have been any more obvious.

JUST AS JENN lacked words to express how happy these various occasions made her, I too was at a loss for a way to convey the amazing warmth and love I felt for the people who had brought such joy into my daughter's world. Large and small, these events had an enormous impact on Jenn's well-being and defined the unbelievable bonds she was creating within her circle of caregivers, their friends, and their families.

Chapter 20

TIME MOVED ON

I began to realize how much time had passed by since Jenn arrived at Squire Court seventeen years before as I looked at the people who had been an integral part of her world during that time. Life had evolved for the Boisvert, Benz, O'Connor, and Rubin families. Chris and Suzanne's young children had grown into teenagers and young adults. Amy and Jeff had a second son, Tommy, two years after their son Ryan was born, thus completing their family foursome. Jenn was well established in her immediate and extended families, and Mark and I were far more relaxed and peaceful than in years past, especially after Mark retired.

But all had not been rosy and wonderful for the Boisverts. There were issues with Chris's marriage that had brought an instability to their home life. All that was troubling for her kids. Aaron shared with me that, as a teen, he loved when Aunt Jenn came over for dinner. "There was notably more harmony in our family when she was around. It was only when Jenn was at our house that all the tension was put aside, and we functioned more like a real family."

I can only imagine this was a welcome relief to him and his siblings and might have raised their hopes that the family would come together and survive whatever conflict the parents were having. But as much as they might have hoped for this resolution, it was not to be.

Aaron and his siblings, Ian and Lily, had a long-established relationship with Joe, the house manager at Squire Court, which had been developed over time from their frequent visits to the group home. He was a jovial, friendly face who always gave them lots of warm fuzzy attention when they were there and became "Uncle Joe" to them.

When Chris separated from her husband, housing became a problem for her, as funds were limited, and there were few options available to a young mom with three kids and two dogs.

Coincidentally, Joe too was facing a marital separation and needed to find housing. After much discussion and thought, Chris and Joe decided that a good solution would be for them to rent a house together. Everyone got along well, and this way the financial burden would be cut in half for each of them. As they began exploring this option, Chris ran the idea past her kids to see if they were okay with it. They all gave a resounding "Yes!" and were glad to have their Uncle Joe live with them.

The arrangement was especially comfortable for Aaron. He told me, "Uncle Joe was a man I could easily talk to and confide in, and he did much to help my family heal." With a warm glow that comes from knowing he had a supportive and loving home, Aaron continued, "Joe didn't take on the role of parent; he left that to my mom. He was just the new, much-loved member of our family. But without Jenn, none of this would have happened. She was such a positive force in my life. I think because of her, Joe was brought into our lives. She was the link that connected Joe and my mom, which ultimately led us to becoming a new family."

I am not sure why Aaron felt so strongly that Jenn was what brought Joe and Chris together, but he had deep-seated reasons for his thinking. He searched for a way to better explain this to me but struggled to find the words. "Both my mom and Joe were so close to Jenn and loved her so much. They were always looking out for her best interests and advocating for her, especially when she was sick or in the hospital. They had this shared bond with her that did a lot to connect them."

I loved that Aaron credited Jenn with bringing a happy ending to the otherwise painful experience of his parents' divorce. It was sobering and gave me pause to hear how my daughter, without words but with a powerful presence, could, in Aaron's eyes, have had such a positive impact on his family.

I was happy for Chris and Joe as they launched into a new frontier of shared housing and a blended family. It was not a romantic relationship; it was an agreement between friends to share the expense of housing so each of them could have a decent and affordable place to live. Once settled into their new residence, they took the next step of filing for divorce from their spouses.

Not surprisingly, except maybe to Joe and Chris, their friendship slowly evolved into their becoming a couple. A harmony resonated between Chris and Joe that was obvious to all who were around them, including Chris's kids. I was thrilled that both of these young people found love and companionship after the frustration and sadness of their failed marriages.

After a few years in the rental, a pending foreclosure threatened their housing arrangement. Challenged to find a new place to settle, Chris and Joe ultimately were able to purchase a home in New Milford where the family still resides today.

AS WE WATCHED all the kids in Jenn's three families grow up and everyone settle into the routines of daily life, Jenn continued with little bits of progress of her own. There weren't the big steps forward like she'd experienced in the early years after her accident. These changes were more subtle but nonetheless significant.

"Jenn seems more relaxed and less anxious," Chris brought up during one of our lunchtime chats. "She sits for longer periods of time and doesn't just aimlessly roam around the house as much as she did before. Is she just getting older like us, or is this a cognitive move forward?"

After thinking about it for a few minutes, I had to agree with Chris. "Interesting! I see what you're talking about, but I like to think she is showing improvement instead of pointing to aging as the reason."

As the years were creeping up on me, I didn't want to suggest that my daughter was getting older too. At thirty-six, Jenn was still a young, vibrant adult, but Chris and Suzanne were right—she wasn't the teenager she had been after her accident.

"Jenn is also much more compliant than when she first came to Squire. I think that shows her level of trust in us," Suzanne said. "She doesn't fight us every step of the way all day like she used to."

"Thank goodness," Chris added. "It was exhausting to battle with her over anything and everything. Something as simple as getting her to put on her shirt was a physical confrontation with a lot of yelling from her."

"I think that once she learned a lot of her daily routines, she knew what to expect and therefore didn't have to fight us," Suzanne added. "She also knows that we aren't going to let her get away with refusing things she doesn't want to do."

I agreed with the girls' conclusions. Jenn had learned the basic daily living skills that were required of her. She was more acceptant of bathing, tooth brushing, dressing, and even being redirected away from the kitchen or food. All this made it easier for the girls, and for our family, when Jenn came home for a holiday or weekend.

After Jenn's accident, when she emerged from her coma, she'd entered an alien world. Both her body and her surroundings must have seemed foreign and purposeless to her. Once she regained the use of her torso and limbs, she had to explore and discover how to function in a world without basic communication skills. As Chris, Suzanne, and I talked about Jenn's continued progress, we couldn't help but marvel at how far she had come in seventeen years. Her strength and determination to rise from such a damaging brain injury and be able to walk, eat, love, and be loved was remarkable. But being the unrelenting "fixer" that I was, I was still set on pushing for her to attain higher levels of achievement even as I witnessed the hurdles she had overcome.

Over the next few days, the lunchtime chat with Chris and Suzanne continued to echo in the recesses of my mind. Was I not acceptant enough of Jenn and the disabilities she had to live with? I didn't want to believe that was the case, but it might not have been too far off the mark. I tried to convince myself that I was better than that, but was I? Should I continue as her fixer, or was it time for me to be her gentle supporter and accept her as she was? The struggle to answer these questions clouded my thinking for days as I tried to reimagine what role I should be playing in Jenn's recovery. Through this process of self-evaluation, I once again recognized that I equated acceptance with resignation, and this would not work for me. This was true during the first year after Jenn's accident, and it continued to be the case all these years later. After much pondering, I became convinced that I couldn't give up on my mission to help Jenn move beyond where she currently was. I felt there were still unexplored programs and avenues I could take to achieve the higher goals I had for my daughter. Conflicted between acceptance or motivation, I chose motivation.

Chapter 21

THANKSGIVING 2010

M ark and I made plans to travel to New Jersey with
Jenn to be with Amy's family for the Thanksgiving
holiday. In readiness, Chris and Suzanne packed Jenn's suitcase with carefully selected outfits for her to look her best.
One of the other Squire staff brought Jenn to our house in
the early afternoon the day before, and we immediately hit
the roads heading south to beat the holiday traffic.

After a few hours' drive and a dinner stop, we arrived
at Amy's safe and sound. We were ready to relax, do some
strategizing about meal preparations for the next day, and
eventually retire for the night.

Thanksgiving was a lively, all-day process that involved
everyone in the household. One of the tasks, crumbling
bread for stuffing, was a job well suited for Jenn. I demonstrated the size required for each piece, and Jenn was pretty
good at keeping the crumbs within an acceptable size range.
She diligently worked at dissecting each slice of bread with
her fingers. Some pieces were rather tiny, which was okay,

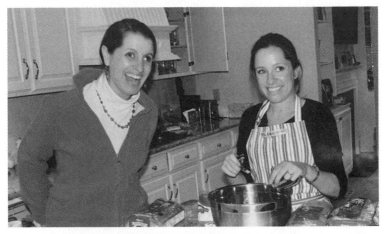

Jenn and Amy preparing Thanksgiving dinner.

but a few pieces were too large and had to be handed back to her for refinement, which she willingly did.

Stuffing was a family favorite, so extra-large bowls were filled with breadcrumbs to have ample amounts for the main Thanksgiving dinner and enough for leftovers. Crumbling the bread offered Jenn plenty of opportunity for sneaking in a few tastes. I was on guard but sometimes not fast enough, and she would fill her mouth with a whole handful of bread morsels. Like a chipmunk who has filled its cheeks with food, Jenn packed hers to maximum capacity. I knew this was not a time for slapstick comedy that would make her laugh. Any silliness and the crumbs in her mouth would become wet projectiles, spraying the whole kitchen prep area in a slobbery mess. I moved her well away from the table and patiently waited until her mouth was empty before leading her back to resume the crumbling.

As the daytime slipped into early evening, the smell of a cooking turkey and all the hustle and bustle in the kitchen had Jenn almost in a frenzy. She hovered over Amy as she stirred the gravy and then moved next to me as I spooned the stuffing from the turkey. The savory dinner rolls were about to come out of the oven, and everyone was hanging close to the kitchen as the magic hour was almost upon us.

Finally, Amy announced that dinner was ready. "Okay everyone, fill your plates and take a seat at the table."

"Can I go first?" four-year-old Ryan called to his mom from the family room.

"No, we let guests go first, Ry. In a few minutes, Dad will help you with your plate, so it doesn't end up on the floor."

"Amy, where's the cranberry sauce?" Jeff asked as he looked around the kitchen island where the food was carefully laid out as people began filling their plates.

"Oh jeez, it's in the fridge; I forgot it. Thanks Jeff."

Of course, Jenn was trying to push her way to the head of the line, but I encouraged her to take her seat at the table instead of hanging out by the food. I held off on bringing her plate to her until the other guests were ready. I didn't want Jenn to be done before others had even taken their seats.

The dining room table, draped in a dark-olive-green, satin tablecloth, was set with Amy and Jeff's best china and silverware. Crystal goblets for wine and water sparkled from the flickering candles set on either side of the centerpiece—a floral arrangement of seasonal fall blooms and foliage. The tasteful setting was no surprise as Amy and Jeff always loved creating a festive ambiance for holiday dinners.

As guests took their seats, Jeff stood at the head of the table and gave a welcome toast. "Amy and I feel blessed to have each of you in our lives and here in our home to share in this lovingly prepared meal which is going to be amazing." Everyone chimed in with a clink of their glasses and a cheer of "Here, here!" and with that the feast began.

It must have seemed like forever to Jenn before Mark

and I allowed her to take her first bite. I knew she could hardly wait to dive into the yummy, mashed potatoes that were dripping with warm gravy. That creamy dish was the easiest and quickest thing she was able to get on her fork and into her mouth. Her entire serving of potatoes was gone before she started on the next item on her plate— turkey. She methodically consumed every morsel of each item before moving on to the next. The peas were problematic and probably not the most desirable. They were the last thing remaining on her plate as she chased them around with her utensils. I cued her to use a spoon in her left hand and knife in her right to get every last pea on to her spoon and into her mouth. Mission accomplished, and all too quickly the plate was empty. Because it was a holiday and no diet plan had to be followed, Jenn got seconds, and once again attacked her food as though she hadn't eaten in days.

As with any holiday dinner, everyone was filled to the brim from the meal but still managed to find space for dessert. We not only had pumpkin and apple pies, we had birthday cake as well. Amy's mother-in-law, Jane, and Ryan share the same birth date, so while we were all together, we celebrated their special day. It was hard to believe Ryan was four and Tommy was already two. Time had a way of flying by as evidenced in the growth of my two grandsons.

The cake, ablaze with candles, was carried into the dining room, while everyone joined in to sing "Happy Birthday." With two people sharing the responsibility of blowing out the candles, we were assured that all would easily be extinguished. Cards and gifts were handed to Jane and Ryan as everyone cheered for our two birthday people.

Conversation and good family bonding filled the hours spent around the table. All of us were caught up in sharing current events, recent travels, work, and updates on other family members. Jenn was of course the best listener. She happily sat and interacted in her own special way: a nod here, a giggle there, giving a lot of eye contact with everyone at the table, and arm squeezes for Mark and me sitting on either side of her. No doubt, she must have been waiting for the next course even after desserts had been served hours before.

At last, it was time to start the cleanup process. We all helped to clear the table, and some took on sink duty to hand-wash china plates, crystal, silverware, and what seemed like every pot and pan in the house. Leftovers had to be packaged for the refrigerator and a few doggie bags were made up for guests to take home with them later—something that Jen paid close attention to. Perhaps she thought of it as preparation for yet another meal. After all these years, it still astounded us how much Jenn focused on food and never seemed to get her fill. With stealthy skills in snatching a morsel here and there, she was definitely on the lookout for any opportunity to grab something before it disappeared into the clutches of the doggie bags or the well-guarded refrigerator. Did she succeed? No doubt about it—she was quick and resourceful, but only a small number of stolen tidbits made it into her mouth before we were onto her scheme and moved her away from the leftovers.

After all the celebrating, everyone was ready to settle in for a welcome night's slumber. Jenn was sleeping in one of the upstairs bedrooms right across the hall from our guest room. A motion detector was set up at the head of the stairway to alert us to any of her late-night roaming escapades as we all slept off the effects of too much turkey and stuffing. Fortunately, the house remained quiet, and slowly night turned into morning without an alarm going off.

Come Friday morning, it was time for Mark, Jenn, and me to head home for New York. Staff was picking Jenn up at our house and taking her back to Connecticut that afternoon. Chris, Suzanne, and Jenn were scheduled to take off on Sunday morning for their annual outlet shopping spree in Maine in preparation for the upcoming Christmas holiday. Jenn's suitcase had to be unpacked from her Thanksgiving trip and repacked for this next adventure with her two friends. They were looking forward to taking in all the stores and attractions in the Kittery, Maine, area.

After an uneventful drive back to our house in Rock Tavern, we found Jenn's ride parked in front of our house waiting for her. Before sending Jenn off, I wanted to collect a few things from inside the house to send along with her. Jenn stayed in the driveway with dad to enjoy the fresh fall air and sunshine while the Squire staff member came inside with me. That brief time in the driveway gave father and daughter a special opportunity to share what Mark viewed as a unique moment of communication, one that became locked in his memory for all time.

After Jenn left for Connecticut, Mark seemed melancholy as he explained the scene to me. "She had a thoughtful, calm look on her face and a confident, happy twinkle in her eyes. As she walked to the center of the driveway, she stopped and seemed to take in all the familiar surroundings of our home. She did a half turn and appeared to be absorbing everything around her, then looked over at me with a big beaming smile. I got the sense that her smile expressed a deep satisfaction with life and all the family interactions she loved so much. I saw this as a moment of reflection inside Jenn on all the deep inner joy she had experienced the last few days. I don't think she could have been any happier or more gleeful in that moment."

I loved Mark's interpretation, but there might have been another explanation for what was such a seemingly magical high for Jenn that day as she and Dad shared a moment of complete clarity in communication of emotions. As she first turned in one direction and then completed her spin in the other, was she seeing her childhood home, and were old memories surfacing in her mind? Was it possible that she was thinking back to her past and to the realization that, although life was different now, it was once again good and fulfilling? I'd like to think so.

Those front steps leading from the driveway up to the sidewalk were where she and her friends had a photo shoot before going off to their prom nineteen years earlier. It was the last big event that she had with those classmates. Dressed in a white evening gown, standing next to her date, Greg, in his black tuxedo, they were aglow with the excitement and anticipation of the evening ahead. Going to prom is a true milestone for teens, and so it was for them too. Two other couples posed with Jenn and Greg on the steps before they all headed off for their event.

Perhaps as Jenn looked at her backyard, she thought back to the winters spent sledding down the slope where all the kids from the neighborhood came to have fun on snow days. She loved the challenge of seeing who could maneuver their sled to the farthest reaches of the yard before coming to a stop.

Other childhood memories of our backyard may also have sprung into her mind. A rope swing once hung from the big oak tree near the stone wall where our yard bordered the woods. She and Amy had spent many hours as young kids swinging and spinning on it, and even more time playing in the sandbox that Mark built right near it. Not far from the swing was where we'd planted our struggling vegetable garden. We'd made feeble and occasionally rewarding attempts at growing produce, but after many less than successful crops, we turned the area back into sodded lawn.

On each side of our house, Jenn could see the homes of neighbors where some of her friends had lived, kids who were now grown and living elsewhere. But during her childhood, our neighborhood was bustling with children of all ages. Living on our quiet cul-de-sac, the children had a safe street to play on and long driveways, including ours, where they met to play hopscotch or draw with chalk. All around the neighborhood, lush green lawns were perfect for romping, playing tag, and tumbling.

And then there was our garage where Jenn had spent many hours with Mark working at his tool bench on a variety of projects. Cutout wooden figures were shaped with Dad's jigsaw before details were filled in with markers and crayons. Cars and trucks were crafted using scraps of wood and an odd assortment of nuts, bolts, and screws. Dad was more than glad to show her how to use tools of every kind, and she was always an eager learner.

The cardboard box playhouse was also stored in the garage. In its former life, it had served as a shipping container for a freezer that we had purchased. This well-loved fantasy home for the children of our neighborhood was decorated with scraps of leftover wallpaper and drawings done in colorful markers. Here, Jenn spent hours in imaginative play with dolls, friends, toys, and occasionally our tolerant cat, Cookie.

Whatever Jenn's reason for what seemed like her happy reminiscence on our driveway that afternoon, it made a lasting impression on her dad. Knowing that our family had shared such a beautiful Thanksgiving together and seeing what he felt was Jenn's confirmation of that left him with a warm, reflective feeling. It seemed to him that Jenn left us for her return to Squire that day feeling loved, fulfilled, and contented.

Chapter 22

THE CALL

During the Thanksgiving celebration, our family reflected on the fact that it was the end of November, and Jenn still hadn't experienced her usual fall medical event. We always expected something dramatic to happen at this time of year. Although her accident had been in the summer, it was in the fall that this peculiar pattern had repeated itself every year for the nineteen years since her head injury. Winter was just around the corner, so Mark and I hoped that Jenn had finally reached a level of stability where she wouldn't have an autumn malady that required medical attention. We discussed how we'd miss Jenn's talking that usually accompanied these events, as these were the only times she was able to say words and phrases. But all of us understood it was far more important that she be healthy and not have to go through yet another procedure, surgery, or seizure for us to be rewarded with hearing her say words for a few days.

Of course, every year I hoped that the fall medical occurrence would trigger Jenn's brain to permanently connect neurological pathways, allowing her to have speech for the rest of her life. When she would talk, her personality reverted to the pre-accident Jenn, and I relished the glimpse of the person I missed so much—the one I felt was my real daughter. I longed to see her again, even if for a short while. And, of course, though we knew it was unlikely, Mark and I secretly hoped that one day, somehow, she would miraculously recover, and all this would disappear as if in a bad dream.

IT WAS NEVER a good sign for the phone to ring early in the morning while we were still asleep in bed—but that's exactly what happened on November 28, 2010. Mark turned over and looked at the bedside clock. It flashed 6:20 a.m. in the darkness as he groggily reached for the receiver. The voice on the other end of the line identified himself as a Brookfield police officer. "Your daughter has been taken to Danbury Hospital," he said blandly. "It appears she suffered a seizure."

We thanked the officer and told him we'd go right to the hospital.

Joe, the house manager, would usually call if there was a medical emergency, but we assumed because it was so early, the staff had the police alert us instead.

This call came just two days after we had returned from our Thanksgiving gathering when Jenn had been fine. But seizures could come unexpectedly. Although we were alarmed, it wasn't out of the ordinary for her to suffer a seizure and be sent to the hospital.

We knew the routine: Chris and Suzanne would drive to

Danbury Hospital and stay with Jenn until we arrived. We quickly dressed and raced to the emergency room, an hour away. As Mark drove, we talked about how she would probably be admitted for a couple of days of observation before she'd be discharged. We were veterans. We had done this before.

When we arrived, a woman at the registration desk directed us to a private conference room where Chris, Joe, Scott, and Suzanne were all waiting for us looking visibly upset. I immediately asked, "How bad was it this time?"

Our friends were standing in a semicircle with solemn expressions on their faces, and it seemed as though they were frozen in place. I sensed they were deciding who was going to be the one to give us the news. It didn't register as odd that they all were in some random room and not in the lobby or at Jenn's bedside. I was focused on hearing the details of her seizure. The pause persisted for only a few seconds as everyone seemed to look at their feet before Suzanne broke the silence. Looking up at me with tears in her eyes and in a soulful voice, Suzanne managed to force out the agonizing words, "She's gone."

The air seemed to be sucked out of the room. My cry of pain filled the space where there should have been air to breathe. "No, no, no!" was all that escaped my lips.

My legs no longer supported me, and Scott caught me as I began to crumple to the floor. Holding me in his arms, he tried to give comfort to the inconsolable person I was.

"Barbara, I am so sorry," he whispered softly in my ear. "We all loved Jenn and know how painful this is for you. We feel it too."

Time seemed to have stopped. I don't know how long I lingered in Scott's arms before turning to the others in the room and seeing the shattered looks on their faces.

Slowly, as my legs began to hold my body weight, I turned to Suzanne who stood next to Scott and me. As I reached for her, everyone seemed to melt into our arms as one. Interlocked in an embrace that encompassed us all, we sobbed and softly murmured compassionate words to each other. I don't know what was said, but hearing their familiar voices helped me stay grounded with my two feet on the floor and air filling my lungs.

We stayed like this for only a few brief moments before the door opened and a doctor entered the room. Gently, he explained the steps that the EMTs and ER doctors and nurses had taken to try to revive Jenn. What he said was a blur of words. My brain was blank, and I couldn't focus on what he was saying. He offered condolences and then escorted our group to Room 17 where Jenn was being held.

There, on a hospital gurney, in silence and at peace, lay my elder daughter. She looked angelic and beautiful as always, as though in a restful slumber. A sheet was carefully tucked around her as if to provide warmth as she slept and keep the cool air of the room from giving her a chill.

As I moved to her side, I wouldn't let my thoughts drift to the finality of what I was seeing. I reached into my soul, my very being, and tried to silently will life back into my daughter's body. I couldn't accept that she was gone. Her skin was cool but would warm when I touched her. I found a place on her neck that I was determined to keep warm by pressing my fingers against it and letting my own body heat transfer to her skin. As long as I did that, I felt I was somehow keeping her from slipping away. I didn't want to let her go.

Mark, Chris, Suzanne, Scott, and Joe were gathered on the opposite side of Jenn's bed weeping and holding each other, unaware of how I was trying to bring Jenn back from the distant place she had gone.

After a time—I couldn't say how long—reality at last set in. No matter how hard I fought, my daughter was not coming back. We had lost a version of her years ago, and now we were faced with losing her again. Forever.

Mark reached for my hand and gently suggested that it was time to notify Amy about her sister. We agreed that I would be the one to make the call, but I don't remember why. I didn't want to break the news to her directly, so I decided to talk with Jeff first, thinking it would be easier for me to tell him and have him relay the message to his wife. I planned to talk with Amy after the shocking news settled in, and she had time to bring her emotions under control.

I called Jeff's cell, but after a few short rings, it was Amy's voice that answered.

"Amy, let me talk with Jeff," was all I could get out.

"Umm, okay," Amy replied, sounding confused.

Once he was on the line, I could only softly utter the words, "Jeff, Jennifer died!"

"What? What did you say?" he asked.

I tearfully repeated the message and added, "She had a seizure and died." I told him we were at the hospital, and Amy could reach us on our cell phones. Then without even a goodbye or further explanation, I hung up, leaving him the harsh task of sharing the sad news with his wife.

Within a few minutes, a tearful Amy called back. "Mom, I'm so sorry and lost for words. I'm on my way to Danbury and will meet you at the hospital."

"Is Jeff coming with you?"

"No, he's staying home with the kids until we can arrange a babysitter. He'll come later."

"Are you sure you're okay to drive alone?" I asked.

"I'll do fine, Mom. Don't worry, I'm going to call Ally and talk with her while I'm driving," she reassured me. "I love you—see you in a few hours." Although Amy's voice was shaky, there was a determination in her tone I knew was her way of trying to free me from concern for her safety.

When Amy needed to reach out to someone to share emotional burdens, her friend Ally was always the go-to person to speak with. She was the high school friend who, from the very beginning, had been a part of Amy's challenging journey in dealing with everything that evolved from Jenn's accident. Ally, who as a thirteen-year-old had lost her mother to cancer, understood loss and heartbreak. She would be a comforting voice as Amy made her way on the long road north to face the disheartening things that were awaiting her in Danbury.

During the three hours it took Amy to travel to us, we all stood as mournful sentinels over Jenn's body. Transfixed by the despair that engulfed us, we spoke only in hushed tones as though we would somehow disturb Jenn's silent slumber. I didn't notice the long wait for Amy as I couldn't leave my daughter's side. Time seemed to have stopped.

I heard a door open and became aware of Amy walking into our quiet sanctuary. Tears streamed down her face as she came into my arms. I clung to her as though she too might slip away if I released my hold. Slowly, after several minutes, I looked over Amy's shoulder and saw the others whose downcast eyes spoke volumes about their shared sorrow. I released my embrace to let her hug her dad who was patiently waiting by my side. After a few brief moments, Amy moved from Mark's arms to hug each of our special people who were gathered in a circle around us.

Ever so gently, Chris and Suzanne began to fill Amy in on the details of the past several hours. Mark and I lacked the words to help our younger daughter understand what had happened. Consumed by our grief, we could only quietly listen as the two girls spoke softly to Amy with all of us holding her close in a group hug that seemed to last forever.

An hour after Amy joined our vigil, a nurse came in to alert us that they needed the room and asked us to say our goodbyes so they could transport Jenn's body to the morgue. The words hung in the air. No one moved.

After fifteen or twenty minutes, somewhere in the depths of my soul, a surge of overwhelming despair gripped the energy reserves that I thought were exhausted and drove me to remove myself from Jenn's bedside. I felt I had to run away from all that had consumed me since hearing Suzanne's fateful words early that morning.

"I have to go. I have to get out of here. I'll be in the car," I said as I made a quick and sudden exit through the doorway and out of the suffocating hospital.

I raced to our car, unaware of the ground beneath my feet. I was running away from the horror and nightmare that the hospital represented. Alone in the car, I broke down and wept uncontrollably. There was no one to see me as I let my emotional upheaval run wild. I grabbed handfuls of tissues that were quickly replaced by the next handful. A soggy white mass of discards lay at my feet. By the time Mark came to the car twenty minutes later, I was a little more composed. He reached for me, and we held each other in a tight embrace. No words were spoken. There was nothing either of us could say.

I had no awareness of where everyone had gone. Mark slowly released me and started the car.

"Where's Amy?" I asked as we began leaving the parking lot.

"She's right behind us in her car. Everyone else is heading home, but Chris and Suzanne are coming to our house first thing tomorrow morning to help in any way they can."

I sank into the seat. The ride home was a blur. Driving gave Mark something to do, but I could only stare out the window at the passing landscape without even seeing it. We were mostly silent all the way—both of us wrung out and lost in our own thoughts of how our lives had so drastically changed in the past eight hours.

THE NEXT DAY, family and friends had to be notified of Jenn's passing, but neither Mark nor I had the composure to do it. Amy, from our house, and Jeff, still at home in Moorestown with the kids, made all those calls and would keep everyone updated as arrangements for the funeral came together.

While Amy was on the phone, Chris and Suzanne arrived midmorning and got right to work setting up plans for the days ahead. They stayed with us all day for several days, offering support, comfort, and valuable input on each aspect of the tough decisions our family needed to make in a short period of time: which funeral home to use, choosing a casket, what Jenn should wear, the day the funeral would be held, and catering after the service. We would have been so lost without them; they were a godsend to us in making it through those painful and challenging days.

So many of the details were handled seamlessly by Amy, Chris, and Suzanne, but Mark and I struggled alone with the choice of a final resting place for our daughter. We were still a young family and hadn't made arrangements for such things. When Jenn was first injured, death had been a possibility, but none of us could bear to think of that. Once she began her recovery, we forged ahead, expecting such end-of-life decisions would be many years in the future when Mark and I grew old. We didn't expect that we would have to face burying our child long before our time came. Finally, we made a heartfelt decision to lay her to rest in a beautiful memorial park just north of Newburgh, New York.

It was important to Mark and me that the cemetery not be in an area we would drive past frequently. The funeral director knew just the place that would satisfy our needs, and he was absolutely right.

The location was well off our normal path of daily activity but only twenty minutes away from our home in Rock Tavern. Once we drove through the majestic, wrought iron gates, gently rolling berms of well landscaped grounds with established old trees welcomed us with headstones and mausoleums surrounding the curving roadway that led to the lot we had come to see. We parked the car and noticed the marker by the side of the road. "Section 21, how appropriate," Mark commented. "That's Jenn's birthday—February First—two one."

Located at the back edge of the cemetery, woods bordered the memorial grounds standing sentry over what was obviously a new section. It was shocking to see the large number of young people and even small children who had been laid to rest within a few yards of the lot we were considering. It was sad to know so many other parents had also experienced the pain of losing a child that we were now facing. So many precious lives gone before the world reaped all the benefits of their talents and skills. The only consoling part was knowing that we were not the only parents who faced such a cruel and profound loss.

This remote section of the cemetery felt isolated from the busy everyday life that existed beyond the boundary of the hallowed grounds we were exploring. I suggested to Mark that we take a walk down the road to the pond I'd seen as we drove in. As a young child, I had visited cemeteries with my family on Memorial Day every year to bring flowers to the gravesides of my deceased relatives, all of whom had died before I was born. It was never a sad occasion for me. Instead, it was a warm and endearing time as I helped to pick the flowers from my grandmother's garden that were placed by the headstones of people I never knew. But the best part for me was the pond only a few hundred yards away, where there were ducks and swans, a unique and wonderous sight for a young girl in the middle of Kansas. As my family stood at the graves to reminisce, I would wander over to the pond to watch the antics of the waterfowl and study the glimmer of the sun's reflection dancing on the water. For me, it was a magical and mysterious place, one I loved revisiting each year.

As Mark and I walked to the edge of the small pond just down the path from where Jenn would be laid to rest, a pair of mallard ducks sounded their alarm as they waddled down to the water to begin paddling to the other side. Flashes of my childhood experiences at a Kansas memorial park came to mind. I shared my childhood memories with my dear husband who had his arm firmly around my waist, pulling me closer as my story unfolded.

Once I finished, Mark suggested, in a soft and unassuming voice, "I think we've found the place where Jenn needs to be."

"I agree. Those childhood memories will give me comfort in this place. It will be easier to let our Jenn stay here and for me to come visit."

IF A FUNERAL can be beautiful and heartwarming, Jenn's certainly met that description. Her services were held at Ferguson's in Washingtonville, New York. Its proximity to our home and location in the town where Amy and Jenn attended junior high and high school made it seem the perfect choice for Jenn's final goodbye. Located in the heart of downtown, the stately white funeral home was one of the grand old homesteads that lined the roadway just off Main Street. The interior was classic Victorian with various parlors and sitting rooms for guests to mingle and visit in before entering the main viewing area.

Once inside, the fragrance of lilies, carnations, and other blooms filled the air from the floral arrangements surrounding Jenn's casket and the viewing room. Before visitation hours started, Mark, Amy, and I stopped at each bouquet to read the notes of love and kindness expressed in the attached cards. The words brought tears cascading down our cheeks as the touching sentiments warmed our hearts.

Chris and Suzanne had assembled framed photographs to display around the funeral parlor and casket. Next to the guest book, they placed a small five-by-seven-inch photo of Jenn skiing before her accident. Next to the casket, on an easel, was a large twenty-four-by-thirty-six-inch self-portrait Jenn had painted during her junior year of high school. Using olive-green paint, she only suggested the image of herself without giving many details other than her eyes. The outline of her hair shaped her face and neck while other carefully placed brush strokes hinted at the leather coat she was wearing. It was a vague but stunning likeness of her that warmly but hauntingly looked out upon the visitors who came to the services.

Chris and Suzanne also prepared a touching video that played in the back of the viewing room during the visitation. Carefully selected pictures and background music highlighted Jenn's life. I watched mesmerized as images of her faded in and out on the screen: Jenn with Jackson in his toy Hummer; a shot of our family assembled on the patio at Amy and Jeff's wedding; Chris, Suzanne, and Jenn in their canned barrel shot at Niagara Falls; Jenn and Chris in their Halloween costumes as Dorothy and the Wicked Witch of the West; Jenn dancing at Sue and Craig's wedding.

As the stream of these and countless other photographs appeared on the screen, they were accompanied by the sound of songs including "Isn't She Lovely" by Stevie Wonder, "Smile" by Uncle Kracker, "I Hope You Dance" by Lee Ann Womack, and "Time of Your Life" by Greenday.

Just as movie producers use music to evoke emotions in their scenes, Chris and Suzanne had skillfully matched the well-known lyrics and rhythms of their song choices to the joyful face of Jenn that I was seeing in their video.

I was so grateful they'd created this touching masterpiece in celebration of Jenn's life. Without their loving efforts, it would not have materialized, as Mark and I were just too consumed by grief to even imagine sorting through a lifetime of pictures to construct a glowing portrayal of our daughter and the amazing life she lived.

As guests began to arrive, Mark, Amy, and I greeted family and friends, who filled the funeral home to capacity. Throughout the evening, I saw people watching the video as the soft music filled the room with a warmth that helped soothe some of the somber tones around me.

Stories of Jenn that I overheard as they were shared among fellow mourners or that were told directly to us gave me comfort. They revealed the many lives that Jenn had touched.

The mother of one of Jenn's housemates at Squire tearfully told me how much she enjoyed Jenn's greeting whenever she came to the group home to visit her son. "Jenn always had a big smile and would come rushing up to give my arm a squeeze whenever I walked in the door. It put me in a good mood, ready to deal with whatever problems needed addressing that day."

A therapist from Ability shared her thoughts with me as she held my hands in an extended clasp. "Jenn challenged me as no other client ever has. Trying to figure out how to best serve her, she taught me to look beyond the normal textbook way of addressing issues with people under my care and be more creative in exploring different ways of doing things. I am a better therapist because of her."

More than one person who cared for Jenn said similar things to Mark and me as we stood by her casket. "Jenn's laugh and zest for life were beyond compare," one of the Squire staff said. "When I thought of all she'd been through, I couldn't help but marvel at her resilience. She made coming to work each day a pleasure."

School friends from Jenn's past also came and tearfully explained their long absence since her accident. "She was one of my best friends, but I couldn't bear to see her like that," one young woman said.

Another classmate shared, "I should have come more often, but I didn't know what to do or say. It was really hard to lose such a close friend. I've missed her greatly and wish there was more I could have done."

Everyone who spoke with us remembered Jenn as a good-natured, positive person, and I welcomed their words. It became obvious to me that both before and after the accident, Jenn had a special way of connecting with people and was loved by so many.

Mark, Amy, and I stood as a proud family before Jenn's casket throughout the visitation and again after the funeral while our Connecticut extended family and Jeff could be seen roaming among guests. I assumed they were sharing stories of joy and comfort as they held others in their arms and listened as words were exchanged over tears and laughter.

I didn't recognize it then, but for the first time since Jenn's accident, I was living in the moment. I focused on each person who visited, and hungrily listened as they bared their hearts and souls to remember my daughter. Throughout the visitation and funeral, the tears and compassionate hugs of others were matched by my own weeping as my eyes tapped into an unending reservoir of tears.

The embrace of friends and family helped us survive the days after Jenn's passing and funeral services. Their loving kindness carried us beyond a darkness that would have otherwise engulfed us. By sharing in our grief, they distracted us from thinking about a future that would not include our Jenn.

Chapter 23

PLANNING
THE FUTURE

After all of Jenn's services were over, Chris and Suzanne continued to work with us for another week to help with two unpleasant tasks that still demanded our attention: cleaning out Jenn's room at Squire and emptying her office at Peacock Alley. During those days of sorting, packing and moving, they shared a touching thought with us. "We were so thankful you welcomed us to be with you to help in planning Jenn's services as through we were immediate family, which we felt like we were. We can't imagine how we would have gotten through losing Jenn if you hadn't allowed us to be with you during that time."

I was not surprised they felt that way, but their words were appreciated and brought tears to my eyes. "We wouldn't have had it any other way," I was quick to reply. "We can't imagine how we would have gotten through this without *you*."

LIVES WERE TURNED upside down November 28th, and not just ours. Chris and Suzanne no longer had a position at Squire or Ability once Jenn was gone. While helping us with all the funeral arrangements, they never mentioned any concerns regarding their employment situation.

In the midst of this, Tom Fanning, CEO of Ability, called and asked us to come see him. He wanted to offer his condolences and ask what he could do to help.

Meeting at his office a few days later, Mark and I told him the one thing that we would like him to do. "Please take care of Chris and Suzanne, as they now have no position within your organization."

"That won't be a problem," he assured us. "Consider it done."

After our conversation with Tom, Ability asked Chris and Suzanne to fill in temporarily throughout the agency while permanent positions for them were reviewed. Within a few weeks, human resources called them in to make permanent job offers. The positions gave both promotions and pay raises to these two amazing women. Ability recognized the quality of their work and knew that both of them had previously been in higher-level positions when they opted to work with Jenn.

Christine accepted a position working under the nursing director assisting with medical appointments and overseeing medication documentation at the Connecticut group homes.

Suzanne was more conflicted. As a college graduate, Ability saw her moving into a management level position in the main building, but that wasn't what Suzanne wanted. She liked working directly with clients in their everyday care. After learning this, Ability offered her a management position at a different group home, but ultimately she decided to leave Ability and move on to another agency. She felt the need to be in a completely different environment, away from the painful memories of Jenn's loss that would haunt her if she remained at the Ability organization.

Most important to us, Ability stood behind their two employees, giving them time to mourn and be with our family, and endeavoring to keep them within their workforce. Not all companies would have been so generous and accommodating to their staff, but this was an organization with heart and compassion that went out of its way to do the right thing.

NOT LONG AFTER Squire Court saw the absence of Chris, Suzanne, and Jenn, Joe decided to make a career change. I could see the pained expression on his face as he talked about Squire during one of our visits to Connecticut. "The atmosphere and camaraderie is so altered now that the girls are gone, I have a hard time feeling connected. I need to go in a different direction." Having attended tech school during high school, Joe was experienced with electrical, plumbing, and woodworking repairs and loved working with his hands. Eager to use those skills, he applied for a position in Ability's maintenance department and a few weeks later was transferred to that division.

THERE WAS A profound emptiness in my life after everyone returned to their work routines. My life had been consumed with Jennifer's care for almost twenty years. Now I had to find new direction and a new way to give my life meaning. There were still some loose financial ends that needed to be addressed—liquidating the trust assets and filing documents with New York State Medicaid. The state was anxious to reclaim the money they had expended over the years for Jennifer's care and wasted no time in pursuing their legal action for those funds. But that was trivial when it came to filling my daily schedule. I was lost and frightened, afraid of how I would move forward after the loss of my daughter.

Art, specifically oil painting, was my go-to outlet as I looked for ways to heal and focus on something other than the inner sorrow that easily overwhelmed me if I allowed my mind to drift freely. Fortunately, years earlier, after training the staff was behind me, I took an art workshop. I'd always wanted to try oil painting, but fear of failure and lack of time kept me from attempting this craft until then. To my delight and total surprise, after some initial instruction, I created works of art that more than exceeded my expectations.

I continued to take this workshop and found that concentrating on my painting proved to be a great distraction during the troubled period in my life after Jenn's passing. I didn't paint morbid or dark art but instead lost myself in the beauty of nature. Animals, colorful landscapes, and plants were the subjects I wanted to study and bring to my canvases. I used photographs Mark and I had taken while traveling over the years as reference material. While painting, I was absorbed in applying colors to the blank canvas and would get lost in the emotions I experienced when the photograph was taken. This proved to be a great coping tool when I needed to escape my pain. I was fortunate to have such a positive way to work my way out of the despair and mourning that came with Jennifer's loss.

THE BENZES AND Boisverts, along with our family, struggled to figure out what was next in our lives. What did the future look like, and how were we to fill the void where Jenn had been? Mark and I occasionally visited Brookfield to join Chris, Suzanne, Scott, and Joe for lunch when their scheduling allowed, but it was more complicated now that the girls were not working with Jenn, and Joe was no longer her house manager. We did our best to arrange lunchtime gatherings, always at the Bagelman, when time availed itself for everyone.

Life got busy, but all of us missed the regular contact we were used to. We quickly recognized that there was a need to reserve time during the year when we would bring our families together, set everything else aside, and renew the bonds of friendship that Jenn had so lovingly forged during her life.

Suzanne suggested, "We've always celebrated Jenn's birthday—why does it have to be any different now?"

Chris's face was quick to light up at the idea. "Why don't we all meet somewhere and make a weekend of it?"

My heart filled with a rush of joy as these words were spoken. I didn't want to face the first anniversary of Jenn's birthday since her passing without the comfort of others. I could see we all needed each other's support as we faced that date on the calendar with dread and deep sadness.

I called Amy to tell her about our plan, and it took only moments for her to say, "I want you all to come to my house for the weekend. I have room for everybody to stay as long as the kids are okay sleeping on a couch or the floor. I'll plan a whole itinerary of things we can do, and people can let me know what sounds the most interesting."

It made me happy to call Chris and Suzanne right away with the news. Plans were made for all of us to go to Amy's house in Moorestown, New Jersey, to celebrate Jenn's birthday. We would make it a "sleepover weekend" with everyone under one roof.

AMY AND JEFF'S house was a multistory Victorian, built in the late 1800s, with a new addition on the back that was completed in the twenty-first century. The open-concept floor plan was roomy and would be a comfortable place for all of us to gather.

Our first sleepover weekend was very emotional as we greeted each other at the door and clung to the dear friends we had missed so much. I felt a deep joy in seeing everyone, and it felt good to be back in the company of people who'd shared our pain and sorrow, and of course our love for Jenn.

During the weekend, we offered each other countless reminiscences and lots of fun stories about Jenn that were shared to the delight of all.

"Barb, I always loved hearing how Jenn stole all the client's toothbrushes at her first facility so no one would have to brush their teeth," Suzanne said with a laugh.

"She did hate having her teeth brushed," Chris was quick to add.

With a chuckle, Joe reflected on how that pattern continued at Squire. "She was always hiding things that she didn't like, even after she got to Ability. Remember how car keys were always disappearing, and we had to constantly go through the garbage looking for a hand splint or leg brace that she trashed when no one was looking?"

"Speaking of trash, Jenn and I were foodies, but not even I would look through the garbage for something to eat," Scott tossed into the conversation. "Man, she could stuff food into her mouth quicker than anyone I ever saw."

"Chris, remember the time Jenn grabbed a scoop of butter off a plate and shoved it into her mouth but then didn't know what to do with it?" Suzanne was cracking up as you could almost see the image flash through her mind.

"Oh yeah, she left her mouth open with her tongue hanging out—the unsavory butter glob sitting there like we were supposed to get it off for her." All this was said as Chris doubled over in a contagious belly-laugh that spread around the room.

Other little bits and pieces of Jenn's antics were shared over and over again, but no one tired of recalling the many precious moments we all had witnessed with her. These glimpses into her life were treasured memories, and our thirst for more was never satiated as they kept her fun spirit alive in our minds and hearts.

After breakfast the next day, we left for a sightseeing tour of Philadelphia. Throughout the day, we reflected on the levity and humor Jenn's antics would have brought to our visit. She would have made a quick U-turn at the Art Museum Rocky steps—no way she would willingly go up them. When encouraged to look at the Liberty Bell, she might have given a little salute—her way of saying she saw what you were pointing out. She probably would have resorted to picking lint off people's clothes during our tour of Independence Hall. Or her attention would likely have been directed at the crowd pressing too close to her personal space and would have given them a shrill moan to clear a path for herself. One thing for sure, Jenn would have rushed to get in line at every pretzel stand and not passed any eatery along the way without trying to go inside.

As our Saturday outing in Philadelphia ended, we headed back to Amy's. After dinner, it was time for all to relax, have conversation, or join in a game of Uno at the kitchen table. It proved to be another late night as individuals slowly slipped off to bed with only a few of us left talking into the wee hours of the morning.

After an abbreviated night's slumber, our weekend's closure loomed as Sunday afternoon approached. Our Connecticut families needed to go home and prepare for the week ahead.

Over the course of the weekend, we all decided to go to Cape May that coming summer. It would be a long separation until we would meet again, but we had a plan in place and could see that there were ways to regularly bring us together in the future and keep Jenn's spirit alive with our gatherings.

THE LONG WINTER months of February and March slowly gave way to spring and summer, and it was time for all of us to meet at our beach destination in Cape May. The warmth of the summer sun greeted us each day as we basked in the abundant light and rode the challenging waves of the Atlantic as they rolled into shore. Relaxing days of sand, surf, and the companionship of our family and friends again helped all of us in our healing process. Our connection to one another made each individual's burden less heavy to carry.

WHEN THE NOVEMBER day marking the first anniversary of Jenn's passing arrived, everyone gathered at her graveside in the New York cemetery to hold each other closely as we cried and reminisced about what had been and what was no longer. The cold weather had us shivering as we stood on the frozen ground by Jenn's resting place. But the chill in the air didn't diminish the inner warmth that radiated within me as I looked into the mournful faces of those who had come to honor Jenn on this sad occasion. I hadn't placed any expectations on them to come—it was their choosing and desire to be there. After a half-hour spent at the graveside, we caravanned to a local restaurant to enjoy a meal together before heading off in our separate directions. As Mark and I drove home, we reflected on how having Amy's family as well as the Benz and Boisvert families with us made it vastly easier to face this difficult day of grieving.

TWO YEARS AFTER Jenn's passing, Mark and I moved to Pennsylvania to be closer to Amy's family and live in an active fifty-five community. Once we made the move to the Philadelphia area, we couldn't justify or feel comfortable leaving Jenn in New York state.

Not far from our new home, we chose a family plot on a hilltop in the central part of a beautiful arboretum that also served as a cemetery. It felt peaceful and serene there with majestic oaks, maples, and sycamores dotting the landscape that separated this cemetery from the busy city. On a crisp but sunny April day, Jenn's remains were transferred there along with her original granite headstone. This monument would be mounted within the arched structure we designed and had installed at the gravesite. An unmarked stone, to be used by Mark and me when our time comes, was also included in this monument. I couldn't bring myself to go to the cemetery that day and witness a second burial of my daughter. Only Mark went to oversee the process. He needed to know that her vault was properly secured in its final resting place and that someone who loved her was there as she was lowered into the ground.

The new location in Pennsylvania certainly made it more challenging for our Connecticut families, but they traveled the distance over the Thanksgiving weekend to be with us at Jenn's gravesite to mark another anniversary of her passing. We all agreed this cemetery was less painful to visit than the previous one. Was it because of the beautiful, serene surroundings or was it something else? Possibly it was because it was further removed from the place where we'd had so much anguish when we initially buried our beloved Jenn.

The trees were mostly bare at that time of year, but fallen leaves that rustled underfoot added color to the gray season as we walked to the top of the hill to Jenn's resting place. As we gathered around the grave, many of us tenderly touched the stone with Jenn's picture etched on its face. Words of love were spoken, and tears flowed abundantly. We held hands, formed a circle and shared a word or two for all to hear. We embraced the moment and understood each other's pain. After a short silence, we placed a Christmas wreath on a stand in front of the stone before we slowly made our way back to our cars.

As in past gatherings, we balanced our grief with time to be upbeat and positive. We formed a caravan of cars and headed to Peddler's Village in Lahaska, Pennsylvania, to browse the shops and have dinner. All too quickly the day came to an end, and the Connecticut people had to get back on the road. There was work and school the next day so departure could no longer be delayed. Everyone was consoled by the fact that we would be together again in February.

As all of us went our separate ways, I left with a warm inner glow and sense of peace, knowing that Jenn's work of bonding us together would last well beyond her lifetime. For us, the world was an emptier place without her, but memories of her joyful and endearing personality would live on in the hearts and minds of those who had come to love her.

EPILOGUE

During the nineteen-year time span from Jenn's accident until her death, none of us involved in her care imagined there was a story in the making—we were just living the life that circumstances had given us. Thanks to the encouragement of a dear friend, I decided to write Jenn's beautiful story of relationships and the impact she had on those fortunate enough to know her. With the passage of time, my emotions were not as raw as they had initially been, thus allowing me to delve into the recesses of my mind and give life to this narrative. It was eight years since Jenn's passing, and my friend was right—it was a story that needed to be told.

As I wrote this book, I learned some important things about Jenn, our family and myself.

I didn't know that in simply trying to rebuild a normal life for my young adult daughter, I had given her an opportunity to connect with her caregivers in a profound way. I never imagined the strong and unique bond Jenn would form with the Benz and Boisvert families. Once Chris and Suzanne brought her into their homes, they committed not only their hearts to the process but those of their families—they all came to love Jenn as one of their own. That was an unexpected outcome, one that I didn't anticipate, but one that was ultimately the best possible result from all my efforts.

Until I began working on Jenn's programs and rehab, I didn't recognize the problem-solver that resided within me or realize the inherent drive I possessed to look for solutions where none existed.

I discovered strengths in our family that were unknown before we were tested. Mark, Amy, and I were all able to rise above our pain and remain a united family because of the common links that we shared: a deep love for each other, courage to face the unknown, and a determination to make the future as bright as possible.

As a family, we consider ourselves lucky to have met the challenges when faced with tragedy and, though deeply scarred, we are still strong and living life to its fullest.

Many of the lessons I learned from Jenn were only realized after her passing. Although language was taken from her, she had developed an endearing and unique way to connect with people. The tilt of her head, the sparkle in her eye, her squeezes and hugs—all spoke volumes. She was quick to laugh, eager to show how much she wanted to be with you, and always a good listener who never interrupted or told others the many secrets she may have heard. She didn't pass judgment and didn't hold a grudge. Jenn was steadfast in loving her people and had her distinct way of making that love known.

Writing this book helped me recognize just how smart my daughter really was. All of us were creating programs to help her move forward in her recovery, but I believe it was Jenn who, because of her determination and love of life, was subconsciously building new neuropathways in her brain to achieve the progress she was striving for. I gave Jenn opportunities, but she was the one who made everything happen.

I think Jenn was constantly calculating her next move and was highly motivated to address things she considered important. She found a way to use the parts of her brain that still functioned to do the problem-solving she needed in her life, and I believe she would have continued to improve and build on her skills if she were still alive today. She showed an inner strength that is hard for me to comprehend and leaves me in awe of her. Jenn was truly a warrior who battled her way back from the brink of death to attain unimaginable heights. She was a survivor.

I think Jenn had many more lessons to teach us. What other jewels were locked inside her brain that we were not able to see or appreciate? There must have been countless other things for us to discover about her; things she knew about herself, but we didn't understand or acknowledge.

The kind and gentle pre-accident Jenn that I was trying to find and rehabilitate had been there all along. I just didn't recognize her behind the more animated and louder version of herself. How could I have missed such an obvious fact? Why was I so blinded by my own ignorance and unable to see what was standing right in front of me? Why didn't I see that Jenn's lack of language didn't stop her from having a voice? Her messages of love and laughter rang louder than if she had expressed them in words. I can only speculate that I was the one who was the most broken from the accident— not Jenn. I bore the major scars from it and although not seen visually like Jenn's, they continue to haunt my soul as I look back on my efforts over those nineteen years spent trying to recapture my lost daughter.

Jenn, who had sustained such a debilitating injury, awoke each morning happy and ready to take on life with energy and gusto. She was never in a bad mood when morning came and walked out of her room all smiles and giggles. She didn't know what she was going to be doing, but she seemed to have an awareness that her people would make it the best day possible for her. This was the person I was trying to repair? I was the fixer, the person who was going to make things right for the daughter I so loved. I didn't see this incredibly happy person or recognize that she now had a wonderful life with no reason to hope for more. Jenn was already fixed; I just didn't know it until after she was gone.

ACKNOWLEDGMENTS

As a first-time author, I needed the support and encouragement of many to bring this book to completion. I can't imagine writing this story without my husband, Mark, who gave me both his time and patience to listen, reflect, read, and reread each section countless times as he drew more of the storyteller out of me than I knew existed. My younger daughter, Amy, was the next in line to edit and in some cases refresh my memory when I had timelines out of order. She also filled in the blanks where I was missing information.

Close friends also played a role. Michael D'Antuono was the one who first understood that there was a story to tell and pushed me to write it. Additionally, he was instrumental in helping to rework photos used in this book so they would be appropriate for printing. Kristen Hinz, Elizabeth Broyles, and Barry Rhinderknecht read my early draft and offered insights into the clarity of its message and the value it held for readers.

My dear and longtime friend, Linda Brown, was responsible for encouraging me to attend the 2020 San Francisco Writers Conference where I learned about the publishing industry and memoir structure. As an active member of various writers' groups, Linda was familiar with both the National Memoir Association as a great resource and She-WritesPress as a publisher and suggested I investigate them as helpful avenues to reach my publishing goals.

My editor, Linda Joy Meyers, president of the National Memoir Association, helped me bring the manuscript in line with memoir protocol and guided me to bring my story to a higher level of readability. The positive attitude she used in her critiques pulled out the best of me as an author.

All the characters in the book were the ones who made the story possible. Their role in Jenn's life was beyond exceptional, and I will forever be in their debt.

The Brain Injury Association of New York State (BIANY) was a valuable resource throughout our journey as a family facing the unknowns of TBI. Within a few days of Jennifer's accident, a representative from BIANY came to the hospital to provide support along with printed materials to help in our understanding of the complicated medical issues Jennifer and our family would be facing. They were a ready resource with placement options when it was time to move Jenn into a rehabilitation facility and were instrumental in helping us choose Hillcrest, Jenn's first placement. Their representative met us at Hillcrest for our initial visit as we evaluated whether this was the location we wanted for our daughter. As it turned out, Hillcrest was the perfect place, not only for Jenn but for our entire family. When the time came for us to relocate Jenn to a higher-level facility, BIANY was again there providing us with information and agencies they thought would be appropriate for her.

Annually BIANY holds conferences where experts, providers, survivors, and keynote speakers come to share information, stories, and new medical breakthroughs in the field of traumatic brain injury. I attended many of those conferences and came home with countless valuable pieces of hope and direction that helped in my quest for answers to the complex problems associated with brain injury. BIANY is part of the national nonprofit organization that provides a priceless service for families across our country.

Hillcrest and Ability Beyond Disability were both instrumental in caring for my daughter as well as our family. Unfortunately, Hillcrest is no longer in business, but Ability Beyond Disability (formerly Datahr) remains a vibrant nonprofit organization that serves families in both Connecticut and New York. They provided the home environment where Jennifer could prosper and grow as a young adult. I am grateful that such a quality facility was available to bring Jennifer into their fold and provide her with staff that gave of themselves so that Jennifer was able to wake up each morning with a smile on her face knowing that the rest of her waking hours were going to be filled with friends, fun, and adventure.

ABOUT THE AUTHOR

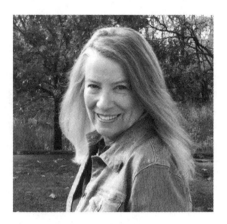

Barbara Rubin wrote this story of joy and sorrow mixed with humor and rage as both mother and advocate for her injured daughter, Jenn. Emotionally invested in this narrative, she had the advantage to write in raw detail about the triumphs and heartbreaks that followed her main character. She witnessed firsthand the battles that come when a person is the most vulnerable, but also saw the gift of human kindness and the difference it can make in another person's life. She lived the story; it was hers to tell. Barbara hopes that her journey, lived through her daughter's injury, will help others understand the lessons that can be learned from tolerance and give hope to families whose path has also been darkened by tragedy.

You can learn more about Barbara and access book club discussion questions at barbararubinauthor.com.

Author photo © Michael D'Antuono

SELECTED TITLES FROM
SHE WRITES PRESS

She Writes Press is an independent publishing
company founded to serve women writers everywhere.
Visit us at www.shewritespress.com.

Crash: How I Became a Reluctant Caregiver by Rachel Michelberg.
$16.95, 978-1-64742-032-1. When Rachel's husband, David, survives
a plane crash and is left with severe brain damage, she is faced with a
life-shaking dilemma: will she be the dutiful Jewish girl she's always
thought of herself as and dedicate her life to caring for him—despite
the fact that she stopped loving him long before the accident?

Loving Lindsey: Raising a Daughter with Special Needs by Linda Atwell.
$16.95, 978-1631522802. A mother's memoir about the complicated
relationship between herself and her strong-willed daughter,
Lindsey—a high-functioning young adult with intellectual disabilities.

Sandwiched: A Memoir of Holding on and Letting Go by Laurie James.
$16.95, 978-1-63152-785-2. After her mother has a heart attack and
her husband's lawyer delivers some shocking news, James finds herself
sandwiched between caring for her parents, managing caregivers,
raising four daughters, and trying to understand her husband's
choices—so, to keep herself afloat, she seeks therapy, practices yoga,
rediscovers nature, and begins to write. Will it be enough to keep
her family together?

Test of Faith: Surviving My Daughter's Life Sentence by Bonnie S.
Hirst. $16.95, 978-1-63152-594-0. When her daughter is sentenced
to life in prison, Bonnie Hirst questions everything, including her
faith. This is the story of her family's painful journey through the
legal system, and of her individual journey of learning to ask for
and accept help—and of realizing that blessings sometimes come in
unexpected forms.

The Red Kitchen: A Memoir by Barbara Clarke. $16.95, 978-1-64742-
008-6. Even the best mother-daughter relationship has its challenges.
But take one that's not the best and add to it a secretive husband
and father and a buried, dark memory, and you have the makings
of The Red Kitchen—a memoir full of humor, grit, honesty, and
adventure that culminates with reconciliation and the long-delayed
coming-of-age of two women.